PUZZLING SYMPTOMS

PUZZLING SYMPTOMS

how to solve the puzzle of your symptoms

For Thomas Cook
My favorite mystery
writer.

Clifton Meador
Nashville
10/11/08

By Clifton K. Meador, M.D.

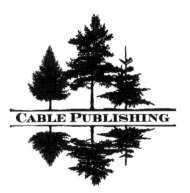

CABLE PUBLISHING

Brule, Wisconsin

PUZZLING SYMPTOMS
how to solve the puzzle of your symptoms

First Edition

Published by:
Cable Publishing
14090 E Keinenen Rd
Brule, WI 54820

Website: cablepublishing.com
E-mail: nan@cablepublishing.com

The information, ideas, and suggestions in this book are not intended to render medical advice. Before following any suggestions contained in this book, you should consult your personal physician. Neither the author nor the publisher shall be liable or responsible for any loss or damage to your health allegedly arising as a consequence of your use or application of any suggestions or information in this book.

© 2008 by Clifton K. Meador, M.D.
All Rights reserved. Published in 2008

ISBN 13: 978-1-934980-11-8
ISBN 10: 1-934980-11-0

Library of Congress Control Number: 2008922448

Printed in the United States of America

Table of Contents

---

*Forms in this appendix are downloadable at www.cablepublishing.com.
Click on Puzzling Symptoms and scroll down to the button.

Foreword

In *Puzzling Symptoms*, Dr. Clifton Meador reminds us how important the patient and their family remains in guiding doctors to the correct diagnosis and treatment. Medical practice is much like detective work. With the help of the patient's history, we create the "scene of the crime." We have to determine, using the available clues, how to solve the mystery. The key clues for the physician/detective are the patient's symptoms.

Symptoms may develop slowly over time. We become tolerant of the discomfort or disruption they cause in our lives, and we begin to accept them as being "normal." As a third year medical student, I found myself losing weight (which I attributed to the meals that I missed), urinating frequently (which I attributed to all the coffee I drank), and feeling tired all the time (which I attributed to the long hours I worked). When these symptoms became troubling enough, I finally had to admit that something was wrong. I checked my urine for sugar, or glucose, and it was positive! So, I then went to the Student Health Clinic and told the director I thought I had diabetes mellitus. He reassured me that I must be fine and asked if our class had been studying diabetes that week. But he did agree to measure my blood sugar. When I returned an hour or so later, he told me my blood sugar was elevated, and I did, in fact, have diabetes mellitus. My symptoms led to the diagnosis and, after I began insulin therapy, I realized that what I had come to accept as "normal" was due to diabetes.

More recently, my wife and I confirmed the importance of paying attention to symptoms that may disclose a serious medical condition. My wife noticed that she developed soreness in her mouth but only when she ate spicy foods. At first, she attributed this to her diet, but she became concerned when the problem occurred more frequently. She had no other recognizable symptoms. She went to see one of our very best clinicians at Vanderbilt who recognized that her symptom could be diagnostic of an important underlying condition, pernicious anemia, or vitamin B12 deficiency. Blood tests confirmed that her sore mouth, or glossitis, was in fact due to pernicious anemia, called "pernicious" because it can develop so slowly that the patient or the physician does not recognize it and can lead to permanent nervous system damage. Fortunately, the disorder had not progressed to that point, and my wife has been successfully treated with vitamin B12 injections. And, her sore mouth quickly disappeared!

I know that patients, along with their families and their physicians, will find *Puzzling Symptoms* to be a fascinating book; one they will enjoy reading to learn more about a variety of medical disorders, and one which will help them become medical detectives!

Dr. Steven G. Gabbe
Dean, Vanderbilt University School of Medicine

Acknowledgements

There are many people who have helped me with this book. Virginia Fuqua Meadows, my office manager, went through every draft and was very helpful in the design of the diary formats in the appendix.

This book would not be in existence except for the diligence and expertise of Nan Wisherd of Cable Publishing. I also appreciate the graphic design of Deb Zime, the cover design by Mark Cowden, and proofing by Vivienne Aho. Lydia Howarth edited all versions and added clarity; the book is much clearer for her efforts. Whatever flaws remain come from me and not from her editing efforts.

Many colleagues and friends read sections and earlier drafts and I deeply appreciate their advice and suggestion. I especially appreciate the medical thoughts of Dr. Nortin Hadler, Dr. Ann Price, Dr. Larry Churchill, Dr. Roy Elam, Dr. Jim O'Neill, Dr. Steve Bergman, and the advice of Adele Baras, an experienced and seasoned counselor for many years. A special thanks goes to Dr. Steve Gabbe for writing the Foreword.

I especially appreciate the advice and case histories shared by Dr. Allen Kaiser. Dr. Alan Siegal and Dr. Joe Merrill both shared patient stories, some of which are included in this book.

I owe special thanks to Dr. Marc Feldman for his help with the chapters on self-inflicted conditions and to his book, *Playing Sick*. I owe a similar debt of gratitude to Dr. Anderson Spickard, Jr., for teaching me about alcoholism and for his book, *Dying for a Drink*. Many friends gave generously of their time in reading earlier drafts. These include James Lawson, Susanne Brinkley, Diana Marver, Patsy Cooney, Hayes Cooney, Rosie Lanius, Gordon Peerman, Jr., Priscilla Gilliland, George Sheer, and Ben Smith.

I appreciate the continued support of Dr. Harry Jacobson, Vice Chancellor for Health Affairs, Vanderbilt University, and Dr.

Wayne Riley, President, Meharry Medical College.

I am most thankful for the loving support of my wife, Ann. I also value her significant advice on editing and choice of words.

Introduction

I graduated from medical school in 1955, a time early in the phase of the rapid growth of the medical sciences. The amazing diagnostic technologies of today did not exist. Because we had little technology to assist us, we relied on listening, examining, and observing our patients. We were trained to use the history or narrative of our patients to make a diagnosis.

We believed an old saying: "If you don't know what the patient has after you take the history, you probably never will know." There was another saying: "If you listen to a patient long enough, the patient will tell you what the problem is." In those days, we listened and watched and listened some more.

Over the past thirty years, medicine has undergone explosive change. We now have the ability to order dozens of blood tests at once. The CAT scan, MRI, and ultrasound allow us an instant view of the smallest parts of the human body. With flexible endoscopes, we can see every orifice and cavity in the body. Unfortunately, advances in modern medicine have led us to believe that every human ill can be seen or measured in a test tube. That is simply not the case. Many conditions cannot be revealed by technology nor spotted in a blood test. Some diseases cannot be seen. But they can be heard. Listening and direct observation have been pushed to the sidelines but both remain essential to good practice in caring for sick people. The story of the patient continues to be powerful and important. It cannot be replaced by technology, no matter how advanced.

In 1961, I entered the private practice of medicine in Selma, Alabama. When the senior partner in the small group became ill, I took over his practice. To my surprise, I found that many of his patients did not have the diseases he had assigned to them. To my further surprise, I found it nearly impossible to persuade these patients that they did not have the false diagnosis of the nonexistent disease. I assumed this was an isolated phenomenon peculiar to an old, somewhat out-of-date physician. That was not the case.

After I joined the faculty of the University of Alabama School of Medicine in Birmingham in 1963, I began to see patients from all over the state. At that time, I was one of only four endocrinologists in the entire state. (For comparison, today there are over fifteen endocrinologists in Nashville alone). Many patients with puzzling, hard-to-diagnose symptoms came under my care, and many of them carried diagnoses of diseases they did not have. I continued to find it difficult to remove their false diagnoses. Both the patients and their physicians were reluctant to give them up. I asked myself then the questions that would haunt me and focus my attention for the next forty-five years: "If patients do not have the disease of the assigned diagnosis, then what do they have? What is the real underlying source of their complaints and symptoms?" In other words: If patients do not have a medical disease to explain their symptoms, then what *do* they have?

I have spent the rest of my career seeking answers to those questions. Over the years, I made a systematic study of patients who had symptoms but no demonstrable medical disease to explain the symptoms, and in 2006, I published my findings and experience with 150 such patients in *Symptoms of Unknown Origin: A Medical Odyssey* (Nashville, TN: Vanderbilt University Press, 2006). The book was written to assist physicians, especially those still in training, to learn how to care for patients who suffered symptoms but no medical disease.

Once that book was published, it occurred to me that a similar book could be useful to patients who have puzzling symptoms or, if you will, symptoms of unknown origin. Thus, I undertook this book which explains a method that you can apply to your own situation. It guides you through a process of discovery for the causes of your symptoms.

Early in this book, I discuss the diagnostic process and explain how the body works. I explain how it is possible for doctors to miss the causes of your symptoms. I clarify some general principles that govern the method of discovery that I describe for detecting the causes of your symptoms. I detail some common causes and introduce you to patients who were able to uncover the real causes of their symptoms and obtain relief. I also discuss some special circumstances, conditions, and patients where this method does not work.

One theme guides this book:

There is not a demonstrable medical disease (diagnosis) behind every symptom, but there is a demonstrable cause for every symptom.

Chapter 1

Understanding the Diagnostic Process and Its Limitations

This book is written for you as a patient. It is also written for families whose relatives or friends have puzzling or persistent symptoms of unknown origin. To begin, imagine that you are sitting with me in my exam room.

Most likely, you are displeased, concerned, and scared about how you are feeling. You are not getting better. You probably have one or more symptoms that will not go away. You have done what your physician told you to do, but you still have symptoms. You may already have been given a diagnosis or several diagnoses, and you are beginning to wonder if any of them are correct. The medications you have been prescribed have not been helpful. You have tried a variety of across-the-counter medicines, but none of them have helped either. You may even have begun to consider alternative treatments such as acupuncture or some of the more unusual herbal or even mystical approaches. The cause for your symptoms, however, remains unknown and you have begun to doubt that you will ever find relief.

It is also possible that you have come to my office only because your family or spouse or friend is insisting that you get medical help. They may be more concerned than you are. But whatever the case, the atmosphere in my office is the same; confusion, frustration, and uncertainty about what to do next.

The process I describe in this book is akin to your becoming your own detective or, in part, your own physician, so that you can root out the culprit causing your symptoms. Before we begin, I want to emphasize an important warning:

This book is not a substitute for consulting a personal general physician, either an internist or a family physician. It is

essential that you have a thorough medical checkup before using the methods described in this book. These methods should be used in conjunction with the advice and guidance of your physician.

I also want to stress that the methods in this book are intended to help those who are ambulatory, that is, the "walking sick." You are up and about but you continue to have recurring or chronic symptoms that will not go away. This book is not for those of you who are seriously ill, bedridden, or incapacitated by the loss of some bodily function. This book is not a substitute for medical care by a physician but to be used as an adjunct to good medical care.

Before we can discuss the methods for finding the cause of your symptoms, I need to tell you how the diagnostic process works. Just how do doctors make diagnoses? Here, in brief, is the way the diagnostic process works in most cases.

First, you, the patient, present your chief complaint to your physician. You tell him or her what is bothering you the most. Frequently, this chief complaint will localize the problem to one area of the body. Some examples are headache, pain in the legs, pain in the chest, or pain in any part of the body. In other cases, the complaints will tend to direct the attention of the doctor to an organ or area of the body. For example, diarrhea points to the gastrointestinal tract, burning on urination points to the bladder or urological system, shortness of breath directs attention to the lungs or heart, and so on.

Second, the physician will ask you to tell the story of your illness and complaints. He will want to know when the problem started and under what circumstances the symptom occurs. He will ask a lot of questions to gain a full understanding of what you are noticing.

Third, the physician will do a physical examination and note any abnormal findings such as a heart murmur or tenderness in some part of the body. He may feel a mass in some region. He may find no abnormality on physical examination, which is quite common, even with some serious illnesses.

The next step in the diagnostic process moves outside the physician's office. Studies have shown that the physician will typically identify a list of causes with no more than three possibilities. He will then check out these possibilities with laboratory tests. In many cases, the test results will confirm one of the three possibilities and a diagnosis is made.

If the laboratory tests fail to confirm one of the three possibilities, the physician will ask more questions and come up with another list of no more than three possibilities. He will then order laboratory tests to confirm one of the new possibilities. This process may go through several repetitions of looking for a test or an imaging study that confirms a possible diagnosis.

One of several outcomes will occur:

1. A diagnosis will be made that is confirmed by laboratory tests, biopsies, or imaging studies.
2. All test results and imaging studies will be normal. There will be no diagnosis confirmed by objective tests.
3. One of the tests will yield a false positive result and lead to a false diagnosis of a nonexistent disease.

Let's look at the first outcome – the diagnosis is confirmed by objective laboratory tests, biopsies, or by imaging studies. There are thousands of diagnoses that fit this first outcome. Take an overactive thyroid gland as an example.

In this case, an excess of thyroid hormone increases the patient's metabolism. Excessive heat is generated by the body, and the heartbeat is increased. Patients will complain of tiredness or fatigue. They will notice intolerance to heat or nervousness. They may notice a tremor of their hands. They will almost always be losing weight. From this pattern of symptoms, the physician will think of hyperthyroidism early on. In most cases, he will find a goiter in the neck on physical examination. The heart rate will be fast and the skin will be smooth and warm. The physician orders a series of tests that measure thyroid hormone levels and actions, and he finds the levels to be high. The diagnosis of hyperthyroidism is confirmed by objective, reproducible tests.

There are many examples of diagnoses confirmed by objective testing. All cancer diagnoses are confirmed by biopsy of the mass. The microscopic picture is specific for cancer, and usually several pathologists and oncologists will review the slides. It is very rare for a physician to say someone has cancer if the diagnosis is not confirmed by a laboratory test. Also, false diagnoses of cancer are extremely rare. The biopsy is very specific for a diagnosis of a specific cancer.

As a matter of fact, you can go right down the whole body, organ by organ, and the diseases of the major organs will be confirmable by objective tests, biopsies, or imaging studies. It is therefore highly unlikely that you have a medically definable disease that has been missed by a diagnostic workup. Modern medicine has very powerful diagnostic tools and the major diseases are rarely missed.

Diagnoses that can be missed fall under four broad categories. In Appendix I, I have listed these categories and given examples of each. You might share this list with your physician to be certain you do not have any of these diseases. Most are quite rare. I will assume that all of these diseases have been ruled out before you proceed with the methods of this book.

What is more likely than a missed diagnosis is the third possible outcome mentioned above – that you have received a diagnosis for a medical disease that you do not actually have. The false positive problem is real and more common than you might imagine. Every test or imaging procedure can generate positive findings that are not true positives. If these false positive test results are accepted without confirming them with other tests, then the physician will make a diagnosis of a disease that you do not have, and the real underlying cause for your symptoms will remain undetected.

The second possible outcome mentioned above – failure to confirm a medical diagnosis with objective tests – is the situation this book seeks to help you remedy. If a patient has symptoms but no abnormality on laboratory or imaging studies, the physician has only a few choices. He will look into his memory bank and search for a template of diseases that fits the pattern of the patient's complaint. These diagnostic patterns are much like templates or patterns in sewing or cabinet woodworking. They are called *syndromes.*

The problem the physician faces is that there are a limited number of diagnostic patterns or templates, but an infinite number of complaint patterns. Diagnostic patterns, unlike dress patterns, are inflexible. You can alter a hem or sleeve length, replace a button with a snap, and still end up with a dress. But if you add or subtract symptoms from a diagnostic pattern, you no longer have the pattern for a specific diagnosis. Instead you have puzzling symptoms that don't add up to a diagnostic pattern. This discrepancy between disease patterns and complaint patterns is at the hub of what this book is about. An example of a well known useful pattern is the migraine headache pattern. There is no test or imaging study to confirm or refute the presence of migraine headaches. It is a pattern diagnosis that depends on a clustering of symptoms. Since it cannot be confirmed by laboratory testing, the diagnosis is subject to error. By this I mean the physician may say that the symptoms point to migraine, but the headache may be a symptom of some other disease pattern or process.

There are a large number of diagnoses that are purely pattern diagnoses. Here are just a few patterns: premenstrual tension, nearly all cases of depression (there is no reliable objective test for depression), irritable bowel syndrome, irritable bladder, non-bacterial cystitis, restless leg syndrome, many forms of low back pain, many forms of joint pains without findings of arthritis, many forms of headaches, painful menstrual periods, many examples of constipation, painful intercourse, chronic fatigue, itching skin with no rash, and diffuse and generalized muscle pains. Many joint and back pains lack any objective finding on imaging. Fibromyalgia, chronic fatigue syndrome, and hypoglycemia are pattern diagnoses that deserve a special chapter. (See Chapter 6, "A Diagnosis Can Be a Barrier to Finding the Real Cause of Symptoms.") These pattern diagnoses lack confirmatory tests and therefore they are prone to over use or misapplication. There simply is no way to say that the pattern chosen is the correct pattern. Most importantly, the real underlying cause for the symptom may be left unattended.

So the first choice of the physician, given no confirming tests, is to pick a pattern diagnosis and assign it to the patient. This works in many situations. The pattern diagnosis will have some suggested drugs to alleviate the symptoms. However, if the pattern assigned is not the correct pattern, the real underlying cause will be missed and the patient will be trapped by a false diagnosis. False diagnoses are very difficult to remove. I have seen many patients in my practice who carried diagnoses of diseases they did not have. It was often impossible to convince these patients they did not have these diseases. Many patients tend to cling to diagnoses of diseases they do not have. There is comfort in having a question answered even when the answer is not correct. That is a major reason that extreme care should be taken before chronic or recurring symptoms are given a medical disease name. Wrong diagnoses generate a lot of problems.

Another problem the physician faces in assigning a pattern diagnosis that lacks objective confirmatory findings is that the pattern often is descriptive but stops short of getting to the real underlying cause. Irritable bowel syndrome is a good example of this problem. If the bowel is irritable, then what is causing it to be irritable? Is it a certain food, or some additive in food? Is it some other substance that is chewed like a certain chewing gum or candy? Is it the social or psychological situation or even the presence of a specific irritating person at meal time? What substance or situation precedes the irritable bowel? A pattern diagnosis may encourage a patient to stop short of finding the real underlying causes of his symptoms. Uncovering that kind of information is what this book is about.

The second choice of the physician, given no confirming laboratory or imaging study, is to tell the patient, that "the problem is all in your head." This is insulting and demeaning and ineffective. It implies the patient is making up the symptom or imagining the illness. If someone has pain or some uncomfortable feeling, who is a doctor to say he or she does not have that symptom? It is arrogant to say someone does not have the complaint he or she describes. I have never seen any physician help anyone by saying it is all in the patient's head. Many of you reading this book have likely had this experience with a physician. It may even be your reason for reading this book.

The third choice of a physician, given a complaining patient but no confirming test, is to find some abnormality, any abnormality, and assign that diagnosis to the patient. In other words, assign a real existing confirmed diagnosis to a patient even though it does not fit the symptoms of the patient. For example, a physician may tell a patient with a known bladder infection that this infection is causing headaches or some other nonurological symptom. I have seen many patients in my practice whose headaches have been incorrectly diagnosed as "sinusitis." All this diagnosis does is to divert the patient from efforts to uncover the real cause of the symptom.

The fourth and best choice of a physician who lacks a confirming test is to tell the patient, "I don't know what the problem is *yet*. I will work with you to try to help you uncover what is causing your symptoms." This is how the physician engages the patient in the diagnostic search and this is where we have arrived in this book. You don't know what is causing your symptom *yet*.

The rest of this book will help you begin to identify and deal with the cause or causes of your symptoms. Now that you are aware of some of the limitations physicians face when they lack laboratory tests to confirm a diagnosis, you should begin to sense how important your own experience of your symptoms is to the search for their true cause. Your physician can bring a wealth of training and experience to bear on finding a cause for your symptoms, but he will benefit from your ability to give a thorough and accurate account of them. For some of you, this search for a cause will be an easy process, and you will find your answers quickly, take action, and get relief. For others, the process will take longer and frustrate you at times. Do not be discouraged that you don't have the answer *yet*.

Keep in mind the overarching thesis of this book:

There is not a demonstrable medical disease (diagnosis) behind every symptom, but there is a demonstrable cause for every symptom.

Many patients have symptoms that are unique and limited to their own peculiar bodies, personalities, or environments. You will read in later chapters about patients who had their own unique cause for their complaints. The trick for them, and possibly for you as well, was to uncover what in their environment caused their symptoms. They had to ask themselves two questions:

What am I doing in my life that I should not be doing?
What am I not doing in my life that I should be doing?

Chapter 2

Understanding the Human Body

Now that you have a better understanding of the diagnostic process, let's take a look at some important facts about the protective mechanisms of the human body. How is it that most of us stay healthy for most of our lives?

The human body is a remarkable self-healing apparatus. Break a bone, splint it, and the bone mends all by itself. Cut yourself and the wound heals within a few days. Eat spoiled foods and you vomit the bad food out of your system or the resultant diarrhea washes the poisons through your intestinal tract. Of course, there are diseases with protracted and serious episodes of vomiting and diarrhea but most of the time both are short-lived protective reactions that keep us healthy. Even the fever that accompanies infections is part of healing. The higher temperature helps to kill the offending infectious agent. Left alone, the human body heals the majority of illnesses that humans encounter. We don't need to rush for medical care with every unpleasant event in our lives.

The more we know about the human body, the more remarkable its automatic self-correcting mechanisms appear. For example, our digestive system makes huge quantities of acid as it digests foods. Yet, we keep our pH or acid-base balance in a narrow range by a tightly regulated breathing rate. When the brain senses even a slight rise in acid levels, we blow off the carbonic acid in the form of carbon dioxide. We excrete the other acid excesses into our urine.

We control the volume of our circulating blood through the actions of a series of hormones that regulate red blood cell production and plasma volume by way of the kidney. We control precisely and exactly the amount of blood the heart pumps with every beat, and we control the parts of the body that receive that blood. In exercise, we divert it to the leg muscles. At rest we divert the blood to our internal organs.

We can tolerate protracted absence of water for up to several days by decreasing urine production. On the other extreme, we can consume huge quantities of water without getting water intoxication. We do this by making large quantities of dilute urine. We can live many days with no food by drawing on our fat stores.

Our internal temperature is tightly regulated, whether we are sweltering in the desert at over 100 degrees or shivering at the South Pole where the temperature falls well below zero. Sweating cools the body and shivering helps to warm it and of course we know to adjust our clothing to assist in the regulation.

Our body immediately recognizes invading foreign living organisms whether they are viruses, bacteria, or fungi. As soon as it recognizes the foreign organism, our immune system sends very specifically coded killer cells and antibodies to eliminate the identified offending agent. This is akin to dogs trained to search for specific types of birds or to bloodhounds who can track a particular scent through a swamp. The thymus gland trains the killer cells to seek and kill only the offending organism.

We can detoxify numerous chemicals in our livers, even if we have not encountered the chemicals before. Of course, there are chemicals that are toxic to all of us. As you will see in Chapter 4, there are chemicals whose toxicity is nearly specific or unique to single individuals.

Most, if not all, of these corrective actions come ultimately from the brain through its direct neurological connections to the entire body and through its ability to regulate the secretion of hormones into the bloodstream. The brain is master of the body. Most of this control goes on far below our consciousness. The unconscious brain is minding the store, and it does so with great precision. We don't ever need to think about the function of any of our organs.

As you see, our bodies are constantly vigilant to keep us on an even keel and, for the most part, within a very narrow range of experience. With some stretch of the imagination, all of the deviations I have mentioned could be considered to be small transient diseases. The body recognizes the deviations, takes specific corrective actions, and we return quickly to health several times every day. It is when the body fails to take enough corrective action that we become sick.

This failure of the body to take full corrective action can assume several forms:

1. If the load of invading agents of viruses, bacteria, or fungi is too large, an infection is established and the person becomes sick with fever, generalized malaise, and sometimes pain in the infected area.

2. In other situations, the protective mechanisms break down or fail to take corrective action because of immune deficiency states, such as occur with AIDS.

3. Other times we lose protective mechanisms through genetic or molecular defects in our bodies. This is what occurs with insulin deficiency in diabetes mellitus or with excessive immune responses, as in rheumatoid arthritis.

4. There are a variety of diseases that attack one or more organs, many for causes still unknown. Thus, we can have ischemic heart disease, glomerulonephritis, chronic hepatitis, ulcerative colitis, chronic pulmonary disease, and on and on down a long list of organ-specific diseases. All of these diseases are identifiable by careful examination and testing.

We need to turn now to another aspect of our brain. The human brain, finely and automatically, regulates most of the body's adjustment to insults or deviations. This occurs at the lower brain levels, far below our consciousness. It is our higher brain level, the cerebral cortex, which can get us in trouble with our health. It is under our conscious control, if we chose to use it.

The list of things we can do to make us unhealthy is long. For starters, we can smoke tobacco, drink too much alcohol, take harmful social and prescription drugs, exercise too little, and allow ourselves to get obese to the point of getting high blood pressure or diabetes mellitus. Just as our unconscious brain keeps us healthy, our conscious brain can make us sick. I do not think it is an exaggeration to say that most human illnesses come from the abuses I just listed. The majority of human diseases in this country are self-inflicted.

All of these abuses of our bodies are conscious acts. We know that we are doing them, even if we say we cannot control ourselves. Sometimes we lie even to ourselves; however, these actions against our own bodies are not unconscious acts. At some level we are choosing to do these harmful actions so we should be able to choose not to do them.

Alcohol and drug addiction are not the same as the abuses I mention here. Alcoholism and drug addiction are primary diseases and are not under conscious control. Chapter 9 discusses these as "Hidden Diseases."

There are harmful things we can do, however, that are hidden from consciousness. There are two real and powerful phenomena of the human brain called *denial* and *suppression*. In the very short haul, these brain activities can be protective devices. For example, denial and suppression allow us to escape from immediate danger. Those who escaped the direct horrors of 9/11 most likely used both denial and suppression to come down those long stairs in the midst of flaming devastation.

In long-term situations, however, suppression and denial can work against us. We can work too hard and too long and not realize it and make ourselves sick in the process. We can live with toxic people and let them make us sick. We can work in environments with demeaning bosses and co-workers and not even be aware that the situation is making us sick. It is not easy to spot when we are under chronic stress and take corrective action. The human brain seems limitless in its ability to suppress and deny very harmful situations. Chapter 5 will assist you in determining whether you are in a toxic and stressful situation that is causing you to feel or be sick.

There are other ways we unconsciously harm ourselves. We don't automatically record the various foods we eat. We don't know even a fraction of the additives that are in our foods. There are people who are sensitive to a variety of substances and feel ill as a result, yet they are not aware of this cause-and-effect relationship. Chapter 4 addresses ways to uncover such substances if your symptoms fall into that category.

It is important that you remember the remarkable ability the human body has for self-healing. It is also important to realize that sometimes we need to take an active role in the healing process. The goal of this book is to assist you in identifying the causes of your symptoms so that you can take an active role in eliminating or confronting those causes. The body will then heal itself.

There is not a demonstrable medical disease (diagnosis) behind every symptom, but there is a demonstrable cause for every symptom.

Chapter 3

How to Observe Your Symptoms

Before we consider specific symptoms and situations, we need to discuss some guidelines for observing symptoms that apply no matter what your symptoms may be. A symptom is a physical response of your body-mind to some stimulus. This entire book is intended to assist you in discovering the precise nature of that stimulus. Keep in mind that I do not know your symptoms; therefore, I will have to stick with general principles to assist you in teasing out the cause for your complaints.

One of the mainstays of the methods I have used with patients in my practice is requiring them to keep a diary. The goal in diary keeping is to find the variability, or what I call the "wobble," of your symptoms. Symptoms tend to come and go, or they become more or less intense. That is what I mean by the "wobble." You will need to observe when they come and go or find out when they become less or more intense. Keeping a diary will help you see when the symptoms vary in intensity.

When you first begin to keep a diary of your symptom's wobble, most or maybe all of this information is still hidden from your conscious mind. Life goes on very successfully without your being aware of all of the stimuli that are bombarding your body and mind. In fact, if you were conscious of all of it, you would be paralyzed with data overload. Imagine how bewildering it would be to notice every single sensation at every moment in every part of your body. We should be thankful that our conscious mind is very selective in what it attends to. What we want to accomplish with diary keeping is to call into conscious memory more details about your daily life, especially anything that is triggering your symptoms. We are looking for causes that are presently out of consciousness.

Dr. Tinsley Harrison, one of my mentors, introduced me to diary keeping as a diagnostic tool many years ago. Dr. Harrison was one of the visionaries who founded the University of Alabama in Birmingham (UAB) School of Medicine. He also was editor of the one of the leading medical textbooks. The book still carries his name – *Harrison's Principles of Internal Medicine.* Harrison was a cardiologist who practiced before all of the high technology was available for diagnosis and treatment of coronary disease. He had to extract the details of each patient's story. I recall one man, in his sixties, who had chest pain (angina pectoris) only with certain types of exertion. The man clearly had coronary disease, as demonstrated by his exercise electrocardiographic (EKG) findings. Since coronary surgery and vascular stents had not yet been invented, Dr. Harrison was attempting to dissect his patient's symptoms in order to understand and advise him on how to live his life more comfortably even though there was no treatment for his coronary disease.

In reviewing the gentleman's diary, Dr. Harrison noted that he had anginal pain if he walked up a certain hill near his home. In addition, there were specific requirements and conditions before the man got chest pain. The weather had to be cool. The walk had to follow a full evening dinner. The most striking detail revealed by his patient's diary, however, was that the chest pain occurred if he walked the hill, in the cool of the evening, after dinner, and *only* after he had a severe argument with his wife. It took all four components for his patient to develop chest pain walking up that specific hill.

Based on the knowledge obtained from his patient's diary, Dr. Harrison advised the man that he could chose to live his life virtually free of anginal pain by avoiding walking up the hill after he had an argument with his wife at supper. This patient still had coronary disease, but he learned to live within the limits of the disease without triggering the symptoms. For those of you with known medical diseases, that will be our goal – to uncover how you can live more comfortably within the limits of your disease. For the rest of you, who do not have an underlying medical disease causing your symptoms, we are looking for the triggers of your symptoms.

Here are some guidelines for diary keeping. Again, since I do not know any details of your history or what symptoms you are having, I will stay with general principles. First, you will need a sheet of paper or a small notebook for your records. I have included a general diary format in Appendix III.

Second, the number and frequency of entries will depend on the frequency and intensity of your symptoms. If you have symptoms several times every day, I suggest you make entries every four hours. If the symptom is more frequent, it may be necessary to make entries every one or two hours while you are awake. On the other hand, if your symptoms occur every few days or weeks, you need only make entries once a day.

Some of you will say that your symptoms are present "all the time." There may be symptoms that never vary but I can say that in over forty years of practice this did not occur with any of my patients. With careful and close observations, nearly all patients can detect *increases* or *decreases* in their symptoms after they begin making diary entries.

Here is what you need to record:

1 - Write a brief description of the symptom.

This can be quite short. "Pain in leg, headache, itching skin, loose bowel movement, wave of nausea, pain in pelvis, burning sensation, or ringing in ears"- all serve as examples. If you have multiple symptoms, decide on a cluster of symptoms and limit your observations to that cluster of feelings. Keep it simple. If you have more than one cluster, number the clusters and enter each cluster number into the diary. For example, a cluster might be "tingling in toes, numbness in ball of foot, too painful to walk without a limp." Perhaps you experience "fatigue and irritability" at the same time. That would be a second cluster.

2 - Score the symptom's intensity from 0 to 10, in increments of one.

Zero would be an absence of the symptom, and 10 would be so intense you would almost wish you were not alive. It is essential that a score of 10 be very severe, higher than you have ever experienced. We want the 10 to be above what you have experienced so far, since later on you will need to try to do things to intensify the symptom. It is just as important to know what makes the symptom worsen as it is to know what makes it decrease. Leave numerical room in your scoring system for the symptom to be worse than you have experienced.

3 - Record the time of day and date of your observations.

Look for "day of the week" effects. Some symptoms get worse toward the end of the week, some are worse on Mondays, and some occur more intensely on weekends.

Later, I will tell you patient stories to illustrate this days-of-the-week effect. One secretary noted that daily recordings of her blood pressure showed marked reductions on the weekend, a rise on Monday and then a steady rise through Friday. She was able to negotiate spreading out her work load with her boss, and her blood pressure returned to normal even after stopping her blood pressure medications. Stress is revealed dramatically through the body, and I devote an entire chapter (Chapter 5) to identifying and reducing stress in your life.

4 - Record what you ate and drank in the time period preceding the increase in the symptoms.

If you find that eating precipitates your symptoms, it may be necessary to go into some detail about what you ate, even to a check of additives or seasonings. Monosodium glutamate is notorious for causing some people to develop symptoms. Red wine can cause a variety of symptoms. I suspect there are all sorts of food substances that uniquely cause some people to have discomfort.

Later, I will tell you the story of a patient who had diarrhea as a result of chewing a certain type of chewing gum. We will spend an entire chapter on unusual substances, (swallowed, inhaled, or from skin contact) that have caused symptoms (Chapter 4).

5 - Record where you were located physically when the symptom occurred and the quality of the air you breathed.

Be specific.

I will tell you a story of a patient who got her pulmonary symptoms only when she sat at a particular desk in her husband's office in his feed store.

6 - Record what people were present in the time period immediately preceding the onset of the symptoms.

A patient of a colleague of mine thought she had low blood sugar and insisted on the diagnosis only to find after divorce that her toxic relationship with her husband was at the root of her symptoms. She did not have low blood sugar, and the divorce cured her physical complaints completely.

7 - Record the nature and content of the conversation, if any, in the preceding time period.

8 - If you were alone when the symptom occurred, record who and what were in your thoughts in the preceding time period.

Certain thoughts or memories can trigger symptoms.

You will want to make your own list of other variables to be observed. They will include those events, people, and substances unique to your life. Be sure to include everything that you take into your mouth including toothpastes and mouthwashes. Later, I will tell you the story of the patient who developed diarrhea from a specific brand of toothpaste.

+   +   +

One of my favorite questions (but only after I get to know a patient quite well) is, "Why did you get sick today? Why didn't you get sick yesterday or wait until tomorrow?"

The question puzzles most patients but a surprisingly large number tell me straight out why they got sick on that particular day. My most vivid memory of such a patient was a woman in her late fifties who had diabetes mellitus (Type II). I admitted her to the hospital in a near coma. She had what is called hyperosmolar coma. This condition occurs with severe dehydration in some patients with diabetes. The condition requires intravenous fluids in large quantities. After she was up and about, I asked her my favorite question, "Why do you think you got sick today and not yesterday or tomorrow?"

She said, "Oh, I am quite sure I know. That bitchy daughter-in-law of mine showed up and talked and talked and griped about everything in her life. I can't stand her. I didn't think she would ever leave. I got sicker and sicker, and then I vomited and continued to vomit. There is no doubt in my mind I let that woman make me sick."

This is a vivid and dramatic instance of the toxicity of certain people. Who is toxic in your life?

There is a lot of truth and much of interest to a doctor in the clichés people resort to when asked how they feel about someone else. Here are a few responses from my patients. No doubt they will be familiar to you.

"She gives me headaches."

"He is a pain in the ass."

"The heartache of unrequited love."

"She broke my heart."

"He makes me want to throw up."

"She gives me back aches."

"I ache all over every time he calls."

"My heart just aches for her."

"It was enough to give me blind staggers."

"It was just a gut response."

"My boss gives me headaches."

Any one of these responses points to a symptom and may reveal a trigger as well.

Let's look again at the core questions I want you to ask yourself over and over as you keep your diary. The chances are you will misunderstand the intent of these questions so I will explain them in some detail.

What am I doing in my life that I should not be doing?
What am I not doing in my life that I should be doing?

If these questions sound to you like I think you are causing your symptoms or illness, let me assure you that is not what I mean. What I intend with these highly unspecified questions is to set your mind in motion to bring into consciousness those things which you need to do and those things which you need to stop doing. Again, my assumption is that there is a cause or stimulus behind every symptom. Your symptoms are real, but a physician can only guess what may be causing your symptoms. He or she will go down a long list of known causes for your symptoms and offer those to you. But what if you are uniquely sensitive to some substance or to some toxic person or toxic situation? The physician has no way of knowing that. He may be quite accurate in identifying the general pattern you have (migraines, irritable bowel, bladder spasms, and so on), but he cannot know the specific trigger that only you can uncover. You are the only one who knows how you feel, and you are the only one who can discover what triggers your symptoms.

Of course your family, spouse, friends, or other loved ones may be able to help you become more conscious of your symptom. Pay attention to what people close to you have to say about what they observe. It has been said that it takes a relationship with at least one other person for each of us to understand ourselves. Medically speaking, social isolation can be a lethal situation. Careful studies have shown that the lack of a social network is the single most powerful predictor of morbidity and mortality. So look around at your social life and connections. If you have let yourself become isolated and disconnected from others, loneliness may be a contributor to your symptoms. Test this idea. Get out and make friends at a church or synagogue. Join a group that interests you. Many hospitals have groups that meet and work together. Observe how you feel in these social situations, whether your symptoms are reduced in frequency and/or intensity after you improve your connections with others.

Keep this in mind:

There is not a demonstrable medical disease (diagnosis) behind every symptom, but there is a demonstrable cause for every symptom.

There are two broad causes for symptoms – stress and substances taken into the body. Almost all my patients who uncovered the triggers for their symptoms discovered their symptoms resulted from stress or from a substance.

The two most common situations are:

1. You are under some stress that is currently unknown to you or you are not able or willing to deal with it. This stress may already be known to you but you are avoiding the solution.

2. You are not aware that you are taking in some noxious substance either by mouth, by lung, or by skin contact. This substance, still unknown to you, is causing or aggravating your symptoms.

These statements hold true whether you do or do not have an underlying medical disease. Just because you have a diagnosis of a medical disease does not mean you should stop looking for triggers for your symptoms. Dr. Harrison's patient had coronary disease but found relief from careful observations about arguments with his wife.

The next two chapters will tell you of my experiences with patients whose symptoms resulted from substances or from stress. You may want to jump ahead and read the chapter that looks like it most closely fits your situation.

Chapter 4

Toxic or Irritating Substances that Cause Symptoms

As you begin to make diary entries, or just reflect on what might be causing your symptoms, be sure to consider the possibility that you may be ingesting or breathing or coming into contact with some toxic or irritating substance. As you will find in these patient stories, the substance can be unique to a single individual. So you need to keep an open mind and look at all of the possibilities.[*]

+   +   +

My skin became my own little experiment

I experienced the uniqueness of the toxicity of a substance in my own personal health. I developed a scaly thickening of the skin on the inside of my right thumb. The involved area spread to the length of my thumb, but only on one side. I saw a dermatologist who tried a variety of ointments, none of which helped. The skin became so thick that it peeled off every few weeks. There was no pain, just this unsightly, scaly, thick skin on the inside of my right thumb.

---

[*]I am not speaking of the controversial "Multiple Chemical Sensitivity" (MCS) condition. The existence of MCS is disputed by most doctors, the U.S. Courts, and by several medical organizations. These authorities claim that (1) MCS has never been clearly defined, (2) no scientifically plausible mechanism has been proposed for it, (3) no diagnostic tests have been substantiated, and (4) not a single case has been scientifically validated.

The approach of this book emphasizes direct correlation of symptoms with identifiable toxic substances and clinical improvement on removal of such substances.

I discovered what was causing my symptoms after thinking carefully about the location of the lesion. It came to me all of a sudden. I had a new palm-held electronic device to use for making calls, taking messages, and recording phone numbers. I used a metal probe to touch the screen of the device, holding it between my thumb and forefinger. Within a month of switching to a plastic probe, the skin on my thumb returned to normal. Either the metal probe or the paint on it was highly irritating to my skin, causing it to thicken and peel. I asked my friends and colleagues, who had the same device, if they had experienced any problem with their skin. None had. I was uniquely sensitive to something in or on the probe.

I want to emphasize that I had been using the probe for many months before it occurred to me that my skin was reacting to it. My case illustrates how reluctant the mind is to slow down and carefully examine for clues to a situation right at arm's length.

Comment:

Although the human body can detoxify a wide variety of chemicals, there are chemicals that are toxic to us all and there are chemicals that are toxic to only a few of us. As you will see in the patient stories that follow, I suspect there are many chemicals that affect only a very few of us. Humans seem to be unique down to what molecules do or do not cause us trouble. There is no universal list of toxic or irritating substances; therefore, each of us must make our own observations to find out if a substance can be causing our symptoms. Diary keeping is a good way to do this, especially if you are busy with your job or family and likely to forget that you experienced a symptom — or even not pay attention to the symptom — unless you discipline yourself to keep a record.

+   +   +

The man who grew two breasts

Dr. Jim (no patient's real name is used in this book) was the subject of a report I published in the *New England Journal of Medicine* in 1980 about a patient of mine who, late in life, developed breasts. Berton Roueche', author of *Eleven Blue Men* and numerous medical detective stories published over several decades in the *New Yorker,* was a childhood hero of mine, and it was a special day when he came to interview me about the case of Dr. Jim. He later featured the case in his 1995 collection, *The Man Who Grew Two Breasts;* Berton Roueche' (New York, NY: Truman Palley Books/Dutton, 1995).

Dr. Jim was seventy-six years old when he first came to see me. He practiced medicine in a small town nearby the city where I worked. Dr. Jim had developed swelling in his right breast. The breast was removed and revealed "gynecomastia," which means the breast was being stimulated by estrogens. A few months later, the left breast began to swell, and he referred himself to me to investigate why he was growing breasts and why it was happening at this point in his life.

Gynecomastia in any male past the teen years is an ominous sign. It usually means the body is making estrogens, and it usually means the estrogens are coming from a tumor of the adrenal gland or from a tumor of the testicle. In both cases the tumors are most often highly malignant. In very rare instances, lung and other cancers can stimulate the production of estrogens from the testicles.

I set out to find out the source of Dr. Jim's estrogens. Repeated measurements showed no measurable or elevated levels of estrogens in his blood or urine. Imaging studies showed no tumors of his adrenals or testicles. There are rare cases of other tumors causing high estrogens by stimulating the testicles to secrete estrogens. Other imaging studies failed to find any such tumors. His pituitary gland was also normal in the imaging studies.

In other words, I struck out in trying to find the source of Dr. Jim's estrogens. I even repeated the studies and again nothing showed up.

I questioned Dr. Jim whether his wife might be taking estrogens, only to find that she was not, and, in fact, had never taken estrogens. So that was a blind end also. I then recalled reading an old case report that involved certain vitamin pills being contaminated with estrogens in the manufacturing process. The machine that pressed the vitamin pills had also pressed estrogen pills, and minute amounts of estrogens had transferred to the vitamin pills. This small amount of estrogen on the vitamins had caused a small boy to develop breasts, hence the case report.

I called Dr. Jim to tell him of the vitamin story and asked him to check on what vitamins he or his wife were taking. A few weeks later, Dr. Jim and his wife Gladys showed up in my office without an appointment.

Smiling broadly, Dr. Jim said, "This was too good to tell you over the phone. Gladys has made the diagnosis that you and I missed."

Gladys, laughing as she talked, went on to tell me that, even though they were both in their seventies, they continued to enjoy sex, often several times a week. On hearing the vitamin contamination story, Gladys began looking around her house. She discovered that the vaginal cream prescribed by her gynecologist contained estrogen. She had used it as a lubricant for intercourse for several years. Apparently, Dr. Jim had absorbed enough estrogen through the skin of his penis to grow breasts, but not enough to measure in the blood or urine tests. Gladys had indeed made the diagnosis that both Dr. Jim and I had missed. Within a few months of changing lubricants, Dr. Jim's remaining breast returned to normal size.

Comment:

This story illustrates how obscure the offending substance can be. As far as I know, this is a unique cause for enlarged breasts in a man. I have canvassed colleagues for years and none have had nor heard of a similar case.

I think there are many similar "single case" examples when it comes to substances producing unusual symptoms or findings. That is why it is essential for you to keep a completely open mind in your search for some substance that is causing your problem. The next several patient stories illustrate how much of a detective you must become to uncover your own offending substance, if there is one.

+   +   +

The diarrhea of Agnes

Agnes was a forty-three-year-old mother of three. She was married to an electrical engineer and had stayed home to raise their children. Agnes complained to me of diarrhea of a year's duration. She said she had it "all the time." When I questioned her more closely, however, she admitted that the diarrhea did come and go, but she did not know the pattern.

She had undergone an extensive gastrointestinal workup by another physician, and all tests and imaging studies were normal. She had been referred to me to see if there was any endocrine cause for her diarrhea. After appropriate tests, I found no endocrine abnormality to explain the diarrhea.

I asked that she keep a diary, recording the time and place of each bowel movement. I requested that she also list all foods eaten and record which people were around when she ate. When she returned with her diary several weeks later, it revealed a clear pattern. Bowel movements came after breakfast and late at night, suggesting food or liquids from meals were causing the diarrhea.

Agnes had tried her "little experiments," as she described her efforts. First, she had omitted milk with no effect. This was a good idea since lactose sensitivity is quite common, as is sensitivity to cow's milk. Then she had omitted all food in the morning, but this had not eliminated the morning diarrhea. We talked about other possible causes, such as cooking oils or seasonings — ingredients she might cook with but neglect to record as part of a meal. Just as she was leaving the exam room, she said, almost in jest, "I think I will omit brushing my teeth."

On the next visit, Agnes told me she had discovered the cause for her diarrhea. She had omitted brushing her teeth, and the diarrhea did not occur. She then tried using a different brand of toothpaste, and she had no diarrhea. Something in her regular brand of toothpaste was highly irritating to her GI tract. Out of curiosity, I asked her to repeat the original toothpaste. She readily agreed to do so and later told me the diarrhea had returned. So Agnes had toothpaste diarrhea caused by one specific brand of toothpaste.

Since I have been unable to find another case of diarrhea from this one brand of toothpaste, I do not think it will be helpful to name it. I have not seen a single case of toothpaste diarrhea in the twenty-five years since Agnes was my patient. Her sensitivity to this brand of toothpaste may be truly unique. I have, however, seen recent reports on television of many cases of diarrhea caused by a counterfeit brand of Colgate toothpaste.

Comment:

In addition to confirming the power of diary keeping, Agnes' story illustrates again how unique our intolerances to substances can be. It also introduces the concept of "little experiments" as a tool to pin down causes. Try little experiments of your own once you know the pattern of a symptom. See if you can make the symptom better or worse with little changes. These little changes can be big clues to nailing down the offending substance.

+   +   +

Diarrhea from a common and frequently used sweetening agent

Rachael, a young woman in her late teens, was referred to me by her mother, who was also a patient of mine. For over a year, Rachael had experienced recurrent but irregularly spaced periods of diarrhea. Stool exams were negative for ova and parasites, and there was no blood in her stools. Endoscopic examination of her colon by a gastroenterologist was normal. She had been unable to identify any substances or stress as the cause of her diarrhea. She was troubled enough by the problem to agree to keep a diary.

It did not take very long for her to find the culprit – sugarless gum. Rachael chewed the gum every day and most days she did not have any diarrhea. Her diary revealed to her that diarrhea occurred only when she chewed more than ten sticks of gum in a day. By limiting her intake to fewer than ten sticks of gum, she was free of diarrhea.

Comment:

Some sugarless gum contains sorbitol as the sweetening agent. Sorbitol is poorly absorbed by the gastrointestinal tract. The presence of large quantities of nonabsorbable substances pulls water into the intestines, and this extra water leads to loose stools and diarrhea. Sugarless gum contains about 1.5 grams of sorbitol per stick of gum. It takes about 10 grams of sorbitol to produce diarrhea in most people.

You may be like Agnes and have your own uniquely toxic substance. On the other hand, you may be like Rachael, unaware that you are ingesting a substance commonly known to cause your symptom. In both cases, the diary method can help you identify the offending agent.

+   +   +

When the offending substance is your prescription drug or its absence

D. B., a colleague, told me this story about herself. D. B. was in her sixties and had suffered depression for several years. She improved on Paxil (an antidepressant) and had been taking it for several years. She had noted that she was actually taking paroxetene, a generic form of Paxil. On her last pharmacy refill, she looked at the pills inside the bottle and noted they were a different color and shape. When she asked about the difference, she was told that the pharmacy had changed the generic drug she was taking because her insurance company no longer covered the former generic. D. B. went on about her life thinking no more about the switch.

Over the next two months, D. B. began to notice the gradual onset of fatigue, a return of her depression and dysphoric mood, and back, shoulder, and leg pains. She returned to see her physician who prescribed other drugs for these symptoms. Her condition worsened with a deepening of her depression. She noted nausea, dizziness, increasing perspiration, and an unsteady gait. She began to need the support of a railing to prevent falling on stairs. She was told she might be having transient ischemic attacks (TIAs or "mini strokes") in her brain.

Finally, her psychiatrist recognized the symptoms as Paxil withdrawal and put her back on paroxetene. Slowly, she returned to her usual state of health. All of her other symptoms gradually went away over a period of several weeks.

Comment:

This story illustrates how illusive a cause for symptoms can be. D. B. had noted the change in drug but did not associate that change with the onset of her symptoms nor did she or other doctors think of withdrawal symptoms since they thought she was still "taking" the drug. The lesson here is to pay full attention to the medications you are taking. If a pill changes appearance, ask your pharmacist why. If symptoms appear, raise the question of a change in your drug with your physician. As this case illustrates, all generics are not the same. It is also important to be wary of counterfeit drugs. There is a growing illegal business of making pills that look exactly like name-brand American drugs. Some of these counterfeit drugs are inert with no pharmacological activity.

Pay some attention to the drugs you get on each refill. The toxicity of the substance in this case came not from the addition of a toxic agent, but from the absence of a beneficial drug.

+   +   +

A woman whose drug was causing a serious disease[*]

A woman was admitted to the hospital with all the symptoms of meningitis – headaches, fever, and stiff neck. The spinal fluid showed lymphocytes, the kind of white blood cells that are seen in the viral forms of meningitis. She recovered rapidly and was discharged home. The only thing unusual Dr. Allen Kaiser could find about her case was that this was her fourth admission in a few years for viral-like meningitis.

The woman's immune system was normal, so there was no reason she should be getting recurrent viral meningitis. Dr. Kaiser carefully reviewed her previous admission records and noted that prior to each admission, the woman had received ampicillin for some other condition such as pharyngitis, sinusitis, etc. The most plausible diagnosis was "ampicillin meningitis." The patient

---

[*] This case and a number of patient stories which follow have been shared with me by Dr. Allen Kaiser, a specialist in infectious diseases and Chief of Staff of Vanderbilt University Hospital.

refused a challenge test with ampicillin, preferring to avoid the drug in the future.

Comment:

A number of drugs have been reported in the literature as causing an aseptic viral-like meningitis. Ampicillin can be added to the list.

The lesson to be learned here is that you should include in your diary all the drugs you are taking. Any drug can produce a list of side effects. The symptom you are having may be a side effect of a drug. If you suspect a drug as the cause of your symptoms, check it out with your physician. If you are convinced, ask your physician to supervise a withdrawal of the drug. The side effects of all drugs are too numerous to list here, and that is another reason why you should become your own symptom detective. What is a good effect of a drug to one person can be a toxicity to another. We are unique as humans down to the level of what drugs can or cannot do to our bodies. Finding your unique cause for your symptoms takes careful observation and a willingness to focus your attention on your life, including the people and substances around you.

+ + +

A woman with recurring pneumonia on trips to Florida

A woman in her sixties was admitted for her third bout of pneumonia in four years. She and her husband lived in the northern part of Indiana. Each summer, they packed the car and headed on their long drive south to Florida for their vacation. Each time they got only as far as Nashville, when the wife would develop high fever and cough. This was the third such episode, always occurring just before they were to pass through Nashville. The woman recovered quite rapidly, as she had from the previous two episodes of pneumonia. She had no immune deficiency or chronic underlying lung disease. She was a healthy woman who was recovering from a curious repeating pneumonia. Dr. Allen Kaiser and his team of fellows specializing in infectious disease spent many hours going over and over the circumstances that preceded the onset of her pneumonia. They covered thoroughly the list of possible causes: exposure to dust, sprays, heavy pollens, and many other substances. They inquired about the automobile. Was there anything unusual about it?

Every time they struck out. They could not find a common triggering agent to explain a recurring pneumonia that always set in just as this couple approached Nashville on their annual trip to Florida. Was there some strange inhalant in or around Nashville?

On the day of her discharge from the hospital, Dr. Kaiser met the woman's husband. When asked about any dust or inhalants that he might have noticed around his wife, his face lit up. The man worked in a business that manufactured electronic devices. It was important in his business to keep all the electronic parts free of moisture. So he packed the parts with special small plastic bags that were filled with a fine powdered drying agent. The bags were permeable to air and thus the powdered desiccant kept the parts dry. This all worked so well that he had decided to use the same powder to solve mildew problems at home. For several years he had opened the desiccant bags and spread the powder about in the summer clothing drawer. He recalled that each time they packed for their trip to Florida his wife shook out each article of clothing. She must have inhaled small amounts of the desiccant when she did this. Something in the desiccant irritated her lungs and set in motion an intense inflammatory reaction and the pneumonia. The man stopped putting the powder in the summer clothing drawer. The pneumonia never recurred and the mystery was solved.

Comment:

There are a couple of lessons in this story. The symptom or episode of illness must be recurring to raise suspicions of a repeating cause. On first episodes of pneumonia, few physicians would even think of some offending inhalant. But with the third recurrence, it is mandatory to seek answers. This holds true for any symptom, and it is the reason to keep a diary to identify both the variation of the symptom and the preceding events.

The other lesson in this story is the importance of another person. In this case, it was the husband who arrived at the answer to the puzzle. It is vital to draw out the observations of someone close to the patient.

+   +   +

The case of the part-time bookkeeper with pneumonia

The patient, another patient of Dr. Allen Kaiser and in her late thirties, was admitted with a temperature of 104 degrees and a cough. X-rays of her chest showed a bilateral pneumonia. Her blood oxygen level was low and she was admitted to the Intensive Care Unit. This was her third episode of pneumonia in a year. She had no underlying chronic lung disease and no immune deficiency.

With antibiotics, oxygen, and supportive care, she made a rapid recovery as she had on her two previous episodes. Then Dr. Allen Kaiser began his detective work to uncover the offending agent.

The woman was a homemaker with young children. She did not know of any exposure to unusual dust, pollen, known sprays, or other substances on a long list of possible offending inhalants. She also did not work in any of the occupations known to cause inhalant pneumonia, and therefore had no exposure to cotton, wool, sawdust, or silo fillage.

Again, as with the woman with desiccant powder pneumonia,

the woman's husband showed up on the day of discharge, and Dr. Kaiser asked him questions about inhalants. The man did not respond at first, but then his eyes brightened. He said he ran a feed and fertilizer store in a warehouse near his house. They had noticed a large number of flying insects in the offices and had installed a bug spray can at ceiling level. There was a device that automatically released the insecticide periodically into the air. His wife occasionally came to his office and helped with the books. One of the two desks where his wife sometimes worked was under this bug spray can.

Neither the man nor his wife had previously connected this device with the recurring pneumonia because it released spray infrequently and because there was always the odor of the spray in the office. The fact that the woman did not always work at the same desk was another variable that made it difficult to spot the cause of her pneumonia. The woman avoided sitting under the spray. The pneumonia did not recur and again the puzzle was solved.

Comment:

Let me emphasize that in this case it was again an observer, the husband, who supplied the vital information. It is so easy, as with this woman, to suppress or ignore our surroundings and miss important clues, which makes it all the more important to ask others for their observations.

This story again reminds us that recurring or repeating symptoms or illnesses should trigger us to look for offending agents or situations. In less dramatic cases, the diary may be needed to find the pattern of the variation of the symptom.

+   +   +

An old woman who lived in a trailer

A woman, in her eighties, was admitted with her second bout of pneumonia in a few months. She rapidly recovered. Dr. Allen Kaiser, having just encountered the patient in the preceding story, was fully tuned for bug sprays. The old woman had told him that she lived in a trailer that was "filled with bugs." She said she used bug spray to try to control the bug infestation. "I just spray and spray and spray," she said with a toothless grin. Dr. Kaiser asked her how much spray she used. "Two full cans of it all over the trailer," was her gleeful answer. The puzzle was solved and this time after only a second bout of pneumonia.

Comment:

Time after time, physicians are alerted by what I will call "the last case phenomenon." Dr. Kaiser, fresh after his most recent case of bug spray pneumonia, found a second case within a short time. In this case, the sheer volume of spray made the cause of this woman's pneumonia obvious.

+   +   +

High fever, pneumonia, sepsis, renal failure, and a husband too late to help

A woman in her fifties, another patient of Dr. Allen Kaiser, was transferred from a local hospital. She had been sick for almost a week and was comatose with high fever, pneumonia, sepsis, and renal failure. Despite broad spectrum antibiotics and intensive care, she died.

On the day she died, her husband, a migrant worker, wandered up to the resident physician and said, "Do you think this here rabbit foot had anything to do with my wife's sickness?" He pulled out of his overall pocket an obviously recently butchered rabbit's foot tied to a string. Then he told the resident that he had been sitting out back of a store drinking whisky with his buddy when a trembling and shivering rabbit came toward them. The man threw his empty whisky bottle at the rabbit and killed it. He took the rabbit home. His wife cleaned and cooked the rabbit, and both ate it for supper. Lab tests for Tularemia in the blood of the woman later came back at very high levels. The wife had died of Tularemia ("rabbit fever") in the pneumonic form. The man escaped the infection because he did not come in contact with the uncooked organs and blood of the sick rabbit.

Comment:

This story illustrates again the value of speaking to other observers. In this case, it was unfortunately too late. It also illustrates how almost obvious causative agents can be overlooked or ignored. Because it was a single fatal episode there was no opportunity for an extensive look for offending agents. The man escaped the infection because he did not clean the rabbit and because he ate cooked meat.

The story also makes clear that even in the face of serious and obvious infections, it is important to look for vectors, agents, and circumstances preceding the onset of the illness.

While stories like this last one have tempted me in the past to make a list of all the substances that are known to produce toxic effects in humans, I know it would go on and on for pages. The list would possibly still not include your unique reaction to some substance. My original list, for example, would not have included vaginal estrogen cream, or brands of toothpaste, or automatic insect sprays, or drying agents in a clothing drawer.

I hope these stories will prompt you to recall some unusual circumstance in your own life. I doubt that you are affected by any of the substances illustrated in these stories, but all of these cases should encourage you to become your own detective to find the substance, if there is one, that is causing your complaint.

If you have exhausted looking for substances, I suggest you next attempt looking for toxic situations and people. Life stress can become so incorporated into your life that it becomes nearly invisible.

Remember:

There is not a demonstrable medical disease (diagnosis) behind every symptom, but there is a demonstrable cause for every symptom.

Chapter 5

Stress as a Cause of Your Symptoms

In this chapter, we look at the role of life stress in producing symptoms. *Webster's Third International Dictionary* defines stress as:

"a physical, chemical, or emotional factor to which an individual fails to make a satisfactory adaptation and which causes physiologic tensions that may be a contributory cause of disease."

Webster's elaborates on the prominence of stress in our current lives with this example usage: "*Stress* diseases are hazards of modern life." In my clinical experience, stress leads the list of causes of almost any type of symptom. In this chapter, I present a number of stories of patients who were successful in identifying and dealing with stress in their lives. I offer these stories to illustrate the power of stress to affect your well-being and to present a method for identifying stress, if present, in your life. The stories indicate how unique and individualized stress can be. What is stressful to one person may be delightful to another. There is no general rule to identify stresses, but I hope that these stories will prompt you to consider the stressful conditions that may affect your own health.

Let me repeat that the information and advice offered in this book are not replacements for a thorough examination by a physician or for treatment of any disease that was discovered as a result of that examination. If you do have a medical disease, stress may aggravate your symptoms. If you do not have a medical disease, stress may be causing your symptoms. Either way, you should be under the care of a physician.

A lesson from a young girl with diabetes*

I first encountered the power of emotional factors in medicine when I served in the U.S. Army Medical Corps at Fort Hood, Texas, in the late 1950s. I was young and just out of residency training in medicine when I became the physician for Amy, a pre-teenage girl with diabetes mellitus.** Amy's father was a colonel in the Army. She was insulin dependent and had what was then called "brittle diabetes." This meant she had wide swings in her blood sugar from very low to very high—going from hypo-glycemic loss of consciousness (very low blood sugar) to keto-acidosis and coma (high blood sugar with ketones). Ketones come from a lack of insulin and are breakdown chemicals from fatty acids. With Amy, these two extremes could occur within twenty-four hours.

I made every change in diet and insulin known to stabilize blood sugars, but nothing broke the cycle of the wild swings in Amy's condition. I admitted her to the hospital every week or two. Even under close observation, the blood sugars went from very low to very high. I obtained consultations from my col-leagues and from numerous phone calls to my mentors. No one offered any suggestions that helped. I tried to refer her to other doctors and clinics, but the family declined and insisted on stay-ing with me.

After several months, Amy stopped appearing at the clinic. I assumed she had gone to another doctor in town, but several months later, she and her mother reappeared. When they arrived in the clinic, both were smiling broadly. I was astonished by what they told me.

---

*This case was reported in the *Journal of The American Medical Association,* 298:35, 1992.

** I repeat, no real names for patients are used in this book.

Amy's mother said that Amy had not had a hypoglycemic episode in several months and that she had not had any uncontrolled high blood sugars. Together they told me about a young girl of four who had moved in next door. Amy had attached herself to the girl, played with her, bathed her, fed her, and become a second mother to the little girl. Amy said that the girl's mother had given her a kitten. Between Amy's devotion to the little girl and to her own kitten, her diabetic condition had smoothed out completely.

Comment:

I was lucky to learn very early in my career about the real and awesome physical power of emotions. Where all my medical efforts had failed, and where no other professional advice had succeeded, the love and warmth of a little girl and a kitten had somehow calmed and balanced Amy's physiology. People, I began to realize, were not biochemical machines, disconnected from the world around them. People were intimately connected to each other and to other creatures in the world around them. I also began to see how these forces of close connection could act not only in healing but also in generating disease and discomfort.

Amy's case is not an example of stress—just the opposite. It is an example of the power of love and human companionship so powerful that they had profound physiological effects on her insulin and glucose metabolism.

Let's look now at the opposite of love and connection.

+   +   +

Lessons from a divorcee with abdominal pains

Mrs. C. was a forty-seven-year-old clinic manager who came to see me with abdominal pains as her chief complaint. She also had frequent headaches, occasional nausea, leg pains, and back pains. She had gained forty pounds in the year since her divorce. She had just moved to town and begun a new job. "I have been through hell in my life," she told me on our first meeting, "and I think all of that is pulling me down. I want a medical checkup just to be sure I am not coming down with some disease."

I examined Mrs. C. and initiated testing and imaging focused on her gastrointestinal tract. All the studies were normal. She was relieved and told me she would get back in touch if her symptoms worsened. I heard from her about a year later. She had lost most of her gained weight through diet and regular exercise and she was free of symptoms.

Comment:

I have come to believe that Mrs. C represents many people, not in the particulars of her life's events, but in the fact that she recognized the relationship between her stresses and her bodily symptoms. I also believe that most such people do not consult doctors. We all have experienced stresses of this kind. We work a bit too hard, miss sleep, weather family crises, meet tight deadlines at work, and begin to feel the impact on our bodies. A friend or spouse comments on our changed appearance, or suggests, "You look like you need a vacation." We hear them, and take some time off or slow down a bit. Our bodies settle back down and we continue in good health. I think this happens frequently. But sometimes we don't listen to our friends and family. We ignore our body, suppress the thoughts of stress, and continue down the same stressful path.

Look at the next patient who ignored the signals.

+   +   +

The case of high blood pressure in a legal secretary

I mentioned earlier the secretary who had high blood pressure

(BP). Mrs. F., let's call her, was fifty-five years old, married, with no children. She worked as a legal secretary for a busy attorney. Her only medical problem was high blood pressure (hypertension). She complained of generalized headaches from time to time. She was taking two antihypertensive drugs but still had poor control of her blood pressure, which she measured daily.

I asked her to keep a diary with daily entries for headaches and BP measurements and asked her to return in four weeks. I wanted her to have plenty of time to get accustomed to keeping diary notes and to begin to make some inferences from her observations.

When I saw her a month later, the findings were striking. On the weekends, her BP was much lower and even normal on several Sundays. Invariably, her BP was elevated on Mondays and increased each day in the week with the highest levels recorded on Fridays. This pattern was consistent during her four weeks of diary entries. The headache pattern was variable but tended to show an end-of-the-week pattern also.

After looking over the diary entries with me and seeing the pattern it revealed, Mrs. F. said, "My boss has a large law practice and is very demanding. He has a habit of holding off work for me until Wednesday or Thursday and then he expects me to have it all done by Friday. It's hard to turn around a week's work in just two days. I feel stressed out at the end of every week."

I asked Mrs. F. what she thought she should do about a situation we agreed was affecting her blood pressure and giving her headaches. She said she wanted to talk with her husband about it. A month later, she showed me her last two weeks of BP readings. They were much lower, with many normal readings. I asked her how she explained having the lowered BPs even late in the week.

She told me that after discussing the situation with her husband, she asked her boss for an hour interview. She shared her

BP diary with him, and her boss recognized a good evidentiary case when he saw one. Together they devised a plan that distributed her work load more evenly. The boss also hired a second secretary.

Over the next six months, Mrs. F. was able to discontinue all BP medications, and her BP remained within normal ranges after she was off of all medicines. Her headaches did not return.

Comment:

The case of Mrs. F. illustrates the value of diary keeping and shows the power of job-related stress. The case illustrates how much stress we can suppress or ignore in our daily lives and how it is necessary sometimes to put our full attention on ourselves and our surroundings in order to recognize how we are affected by stress. Best of all, the case shows a method for dealing with job-related stress. Fortunately, Mrs. F. had an understanding and caring boss who valued his outstanding legal secretary.

Sometimes a diagnosis of a medical disease can be misleading and divert attention away from stress, as in the next patient.

+   +   +

The case of Lonzo C., whose stress was mistaken for a disease he didn't have

Lonzo C. was a thirty-eight-year-old truck driver. He told me he had been diagnosed with hypoglycemia (low blood sugar). He had been told to avoid all sweets and to eat six meals a day, all high in protein. He had been following the diet for several weeks with no improvement in his symptoms.

I asked him about the symptoms. He told me he was anxious, jittery in his stomach, couldn't sleep soundly, had dry mouth a lot, and worried all the time. He denied feeling depressed. His routine workup and several blood sugar tests were all normal.

I asked him to keep a diary of his symptoms and to record food he ate and other factors, such as who was with him when he had the symptoms.

When I saw him a few weeks later, he told me, "You know, if I hadn't been told I had low blood sugar, I would swear my troubles are coming from my new driving partner and that wife of mine."

His new partner, Lonzo said, had been assigned to him by his boss. Lonzo was a devoutly religious man and could not abide profanity or "womanizing." His new partner cursed all the time and whenever they stopped at a truck stop, the partner tried to put the make on the waitresses and draw Lonzo into his seductions. Lonzo's diary indicated his symptoms were more acute when he spent time on the road with his driving partner. Time at home was also not ideal for Lonzo because marital relations had worsened. His wife had been an unusually "dutiful" wife early in the marriage. She had stayed home, cleaned the house, cooked, and was everything Lonzo dreamed of in a wife. Then she had changed. She had returned to school, begun spending more time with her friends, and recently had found a job of her own. Lonzo told me that between his womanizing partner and his newly independent wife, his life had "come apart." His symptom diary had verified for him that these stresses were having an effect on him physically.

I saw Lonzo C. from time to time. He succeeded in persuading his boss to restore his original driving partner, and he began having long conversations with his wife that improved their relationship. In a few months, almost all of his symptoms went away. Lonzo C. told me he was enjoying candy bars again with no symptoms.

Comment:

A diagnosis of hypoglycemia, in my experience, may be the

most misleading of all false diagnoses. Lonzo C. is an example of that problem. The diagnosis diverted him from finding the true causes of his symptoms.

True documented spontaneous hypoglycemia is extremely rare. I have had only three patients with documented true spontaneous hypoglycemia in over fifty years of clinical practice. (To underscore its rarity, please keep in mind that my practice was largely one of the endocrine diseases, where people with hypoglycemia usually end up.) Two of the patients had insulin-secreting tumors of the pancreas. The third patient surreptitiously injected herself with insulin, creating a diagnostic nightmare, which was not ended until an intern found her insulin syringe in her bedside table. She came dangerously close to risking exploratory surgery of her pancreas.

Of course, there are many people with diabetes mellitus who become hypoglycemic from taking insulin or oral agents. Hypoglycemia is quite common among people taking these agents. Prolonged fasting in alcoholics can produce hypoglycemia, and there are rare conditions in childhood of spontaneous hypoglycemia. But spontaneous hypoglycemia in adults is extremely rare.

Despite its rarity, however, hypoglycemia is an extraordinarily popular subject. In a recent Google search, for example, I found 3,600,000 entries for hypoglycemia. There are many associations and organizations devoted to the term. The kind of so-called hypoglycemia that draws so much attention and misdirection is what is labeled "reactive hypoglycemia." If you eat a lot of sugar, the blood sugar will rise and then fall. The fall will sometimes drop below the baseline value. This dip has been erroneously labeled "hypoglycemia."

I do not doubt for a second that people labeled "hypoglycemic" are truly suffering in some way. They are having symptoms of varied sorts but the label is usually misleading. If you have been diagnosed as hypoglycemic, but blood sugar tests do not support the diagnosis, I urge you to look beyond that label to the events and environment of your life. Something is causing your symptom, but it is highly unlikely the cause is hypoglycemia.

Here is another story that illustrates the difficulty in removing a diagnosis of hypoglycemia.

+   +   +

The woman who thought she was hypoglycemic

A woman in her early thirties came to see a colleague of mine with a diagnosis of hypoglycemia. Being a thorough endocrinologist, he set out to draw a blood sugar every the woman had her symptoms. He obtained over a dozen blood sugars, and all were normal. Her symptoms were primarily ones of anxiousness and anxiety, jitteriness, weak feelings, and sweatiness. She had difficulty sleeping. She denied depression and did not appear depressed to my colleague.

In a follow-up appointment, my colleague carefully went over every normal blood sugar. He also reviewed her symptoms at the time each blood sugar was measured, but he still could not find a clear cause for her symptoms. The woman was very irritated with him. "I don't care what you say," she said as she stood to walk out of his office. "I still have hypoglycemia." She refused any more discussion of her symptoms.

Many months later, however, my colleague got a phone call from the woman. "I just wanted to call and tell you I am cured," she said.

"That's great," my colleague said, "How did it come about?"

"I got a divorce," she said. All of her symptoms went away with the divorce.

Comment:

This story illustrates two very strong lessons. First, a diagnosis of "hypoglycemia" in nearly all cases hides or obscures the real causes of the symptoms. The symptoms are real. The diagnosis is false. The label prevents further efforts to find the real causes.

The second lesson is that many people endure toxic relationships. These relationships can produce a large variety of physical symptoms. Careful observations of your life, your relationships, and your environment can uncover the toxicities in your life. It may not be necessary to get a divorce to escape the symptoms but it is necessary to uncover their true causes before you can begin to cure them. Don't let false diagnoses prevent you from knowing the truth. Sometimes we jump to diagnoses too soon. While it is often comforting to have a name for our problems, it is false comfort, in the long run, if it is the wrong name.

"You will know the truth, and the truth will make you free." (John 8:32)

Sometimes stresses can be very complex and difficult to unravel, as they were for the next patient.

+   +   +

A secretary with a complicated work situation

Cathy was an unmarried twenty-eight-year-old secretary. She complained of diarrhea of a three-year duration and a slow weight loss of fifteen pounds. She had been hospitalized twice before consulting me. On the first admission, she was told she had gall bladder disease, and her gall bladder was removed. The diarrhea continued. On the second hospitalization, she had an extensive workup for gastrointestinal malabsorption, including a small bowel biopsy. She changed physicians and was told by the new doctor that she had either ulcerative colitis or Crohn's disease. On her first visit with me, she indicated that she had read extensively about both diseases and was considering a partial or total removal of her colon. We scheduled some tests and lab work and agreed to meet again after I received the results.

At our next meeting, we discussed the fact that a review of her outside radiological studies and test results together with a repeat barium enema, an endoscopic examination of her colon, and tests for blood in her stools were all negative. I advised her to delay surgery, suggested she begin keeping a symptom diary, and asked a few questions about her home and work conditions. She admitted to having some difficulties with her boss, going so far as to say that she hated him. "But none of that has anything to do with my colitis," she insisted.

I suggested Cathy keep a detailed diary and record each stool, its place and time of occurrence, its relation to meals, and the content of each meal. For two weeks, Cathy focused on foods as the cause of her symptoms. She even tried eliminating milk and a variety of other foods, but these changes did not reduce the diarrhea. She recorded less diarrhea on the weekends and more during the week. After seeing no correlation between what she ate and her symptoms, she began to see a connection between her diarrhea and the intensity of her conflict with her boss. The conflict revolved around her need for a job so she could continue her night college work and her knowledge of her boss' embezzling. She feared that she would lose her job and income if she reported him, and also feared his threats to involve her in his crime. If she did not report him however, she would continue to feel guilty and unworthy.

After several months of indecision and physical suffering, Cathy quit her job and reported her boss to the president of the company. Within a month of taking action the diarrhea ceased and she remained free of it over the year I continued to hear from her.

Comment:

Once again, a false diagnosis diverted attention away from the real cause of symptoms. In this case, it led to unnecessary gall bladder surgery. The power of a false diagnosis cannot be overemphasized.

Cathy's story underscores the importance of looking behind the label you may have been given to what is going on in your life. Even if Cathy had suffered documented colitis, diary keeping would still have had value. The question for her then would have been, "What in your life is aggravating the symptoms of your colitis?" Medical diseases are often greatly aggravated by stress, so keep track of your symptoms and when they "wobble." Even if you have a medical disease, you may be able to reduce the severity of your symptoms by identifying and eliminating stresses in your life.

In Cathy's case, the situation was complex and unique. I doubt if there are many embezzling bosses causing diarrhea in their secretaries. The point here is that each of us is unique, and we all have our unique stresses and responses to stress.

What am I doing in my life that I should not be doing?
What am I not doing in my life that I should be doing?

Look at these two questions carefully; notice that both use highly unspecified language. "What am I doing?" could apply to almost anything in your entire life. The general nature of the wording is what makes the question so powerful. It prompts your mind to search every aspect of your life to find something you can stop doing. The same power flows from "What am I *not* doing?" Let these general questions soak into the deepest parts of your mind and spirit. Ask yourself these questions each time you make an entry in your diary. You will find your own specific answers.

Chapter 6

A Diagnosis Can Be a Barrier to Finding the Real Cause of Symptoms

In the previous chapter, I told you about two people whose false diagnosis of hypoglycemia interfered with their ability to recognize stress as the true cause of their symptoms. It may sound strange, but sometimes a diagnosis, even when correct, can be a barrier to finding the real causes for symptoms.

Let me explain. Assume there are two hypothetical patients. One patient has chronic lung disease and the other has no lung disease. Both are coughing. The diary records of both revealed that the coughing occurs mainly in a dusty room filled with mildew. The coughing of both improves after the room is thoroughly cleaned and aired. If the diagnosis "chronic lung disease" had been accepted as the sole cause of all coughing in the first patient, then the real cause would have been missed. No matter how serious or dramatic symptoms of a medical disease may be, there is always the possibility that some environmental factor is playing an aggravating or causative role.

A medical diagnosis, even when accurate, does not necessarily explain all symptoms. People with medical diseases also have toxic relationships, eat toxic foods or additives, breathe unclean air, and have all of the harmful substances and stresses of those without a medical disease. Certainly medical diseases produce symptoms from the internal dysfunctions of the disease but these patients are equally, and sometimes more, susceptible to aggravating environmental factors. You may recall the patient of Dr. Tinsley Harrison in Chapter 3, who had coronary disease but got symptoms walking up a specific hill, after dinner, but only after he'd had an argument with his wife. Diary keeping is just as important for those of you with a medical disease as it is for those of you who do not have a medical disease.

Remember this: There are only a limited number of templates or patterns of medical diseases. However, there are an infinite number of environmental factors that can cause your unique symptoms. This is true whether you have a medical disease or not. A diagnosis of a medical disease should not stop your search for aggravating factors.

While a correct medical diagnosis can be a barrier to uncovering the cause of a symptom, the most difficult barrier to helping people with puzzling symptoms is the presence of an incorrect diagnosis. By that I mean a diagnosis of a disease that is not present. In this chapter, I will examine this problem in more detail and take a look at three diagnoses I find especially troubling.

In the introduction, I mentioned my very early experience of covering the practice of a senior partner and discovering that many of his patients did not have the disease he had assigned them. Over the years, I have discovered this is not an uncommon experience. I have met many people who carried diagnoses of diseases they did not have.

Most of us derive some comfort from being able to name our fears and our problems. Not knowing what is in a darkened room is often more frightening than hearing what it is, even if we have no sure proof. When we are frightened by symptoms or are in pain, we tend to trust the authority — whether it is a doctor or an Internet site that offers relief with a diagnosis. Being able to name a disease and talk about how it occurs and what it does to the body possibly increases a person's sense of control over his puzzling symptoms. They are not a puzzle any longer; they fit a pattern that has a name. And beware to the expert who comes along and tips the table over, spilling the pieces into a jumbled puzzle once more. Sometimes people become so obsessed with their nonexistent diseases, they reject any discussion as heresy.

In my book, *Symptoms of Unknown Origin*, I reported my findings on seventy-eight patients who had multiple symptoms but no demonstrable medical disease. I saw these patients over a number of years and did extensive workups on all of them, looking for medical diseases. All of my tests and imaging studies were normal in these seventy-eight patients. The majority of the patients (forty-two out of seventy-eight) carried diagnoses of nonexistent diseases. Some patients had two or more false diagnoses.

Here is a list of the diagnoses of diseases in these forty-two patients which were *not* found after extensive testing.

diabetes mellitus (two patients)
duodenal ulcer (two patients)
hyperthyroidism (two patients)
hypoglycemia (four patients)
malignant lipoma
multiple allergies (two patients)
ovarian failure
sinusitis
ulcerative colitis (two patients)
acromegaly
congenital heart disease
hiatus hernia (three patients)
hypertension
hypothyroidism
rheumatoid arthritis
uterine tumor
abscesses of teeth
bladder obstruction (three patients)
cerebral aneurysm
coronary artery disease
"detaching" retina
heart failure

lymphoma
migraine headaches
stroke (two patients)
thrombophlebitis
thyroiditis (two patients)

Of these forty-two patients, I was not able to convince twenty-five that they did not have the named disease. These patients continued to insist they had the disease. I was able to convince seventeen of the patients that the disease they thought they had was not present. The false label was more powerful to more patients who carry it than any evidence or argument or authority against it. That is a phenomenon that still perplexes and troubles me today. There is an old saying in medicine: "Once a doctor and a patient agree on a diagnosis of a chronic condition, the condition becomes incurable." My experience with the twenty-five patients who refused to drop their false diagnoses confirms that saying. To me, it is still a challenge to discover how to reach patients who will not surrender their false diagnoses and attempt to uncover the true causes of these sometimes very painful symptoms.

Of all the false diagnoses I have encountered, there are three that seem particularly difficult to persuade people to give up. Many people with these diagnoses become highly defensive, even strident, and insist that they have their disease, despite all the evidence to the contrary.

These three most stubbornly defended false labels in my experience are: fibromyalgia, hypoglycemia, and chronic fatigue syndrome.

Recently, out of curiosity, and even though I am now retired from practice, I entered these terms into the Google search engine and found the following number of sites listed for each: chronic fatigue syndrome, 2,140,000 sites; fibromyalgia, 6,280,000 sites;

hypoglycemia, 3,620,000 sites. Just for comparison I also entered coronary artery disease (which kills more Americans each year than any other disease). My search produced 2,380,000 sites. Rheumatoid arthritis, another common disease which can be diagnosed in laboratory studies, produced 2,220,000 sites.

Still curious, I compared the symptoms listed for fibromyalgia, chronic fatigue syndrome, and hypoglycemia by the *Mayo Clinic Bulletins* and the Hypoglycemia Foundation. I found the sixteen symptoms listed below to be common to all three conditions. The overlap in symptoms is huge, and there is no specific test, biopsy, or imaging study to define fibromyalgia or chronic fatigue syndrome. However, anyone with several of these symptoms who goes to the Internet for help might find misleading "proof" that he or she has a named condition.

The sixteen symptoms common to fibromyalgia, chronic fatigue syndrome, and hypoglycemia are:

chronic fatigue
impaired memory
anxiety
muscle pains
headaches
unrefreshing sleep
abdominal pains
bloating
chest pain
stiffness
diarrhea
depression
tingling sensations in skin
difficulty concentrating
dry eyes and mouth
dizziness

Do not misunderstand me. I am not arguing that people who have been labeled with chronic fatigue syndrome, fibromyalgia, or hypoglycemia are faking it. People who have been referred to me with these labels are very uncomfortable and suffer a lot. I see no value in naming the conditions when there is no specificity to the symptoms, no specific tests, and most important, no specific or effective treatment.

I believe that patients who carry these labels would benefit, instead, from recognition of their symptoms as real and puzzling. Then it will be possible for doctor and patient to attempt to tease out the underlying causes for the symptoms. I firmly endorse the use of diary keeping to help these patients find triggers for their complaints as a means to eliminate them. As it stands now, these people diagnosed with these conditions accept a label of a disease that cannot be confirmed and for which there is no treatment. These labels bring to an abrupt halt any search for underlying causes of the symptoms. Once labeled, the person is trapped for life. What value is a label of a disease if it leads nowhere and cannot be confirmed? Why not try to find the underlying triggers to their symptoms?

+ + +

Some advice for family members

If someone in your family has been diagnosed with one of these conditions, then you might be able to assist them in finding correlations with triggers and identifying situations where their symptoms wobble or become more severe. Family members sometimes have more success pointing out triggering circumstances than doctors do. Do not waste your time in trying to convince your wife, husband, brother, mother, aunt, or uncle that they do not have the named conditions. In the long run, try to work on your relationship with the person. If you let the label of the disease get between you and the person, the relationship will eventually suffer or come apart.

One final suggestion: It does no good to ask repeatedly how someone with these conditions is feeling. Doing so may even remind them of their symptoms in periods when they are relatively comfortable. You did not cause the problems, you cannot cure the problems, and you cannot control the problems. You may, however, contribute to the problem by paying too much attention to it.

Let the patient take the lead in reporting the symptom, and make your job the work of helping the person recognize the circumstances when he or she experiences it. Turning yourself into an observer of this kind can coach the patient to become a more accurate reporter. Family members can learn in this way how to empower, rather than rescue, the patient.

When these coaching approaches fail, there is a paradoxical approach best summed up, "An ignored behavior eventually extinguishes itself." I have seen this work in families where all have quietly agreed to ignore the insistent complaints of the family member. I have more to say on this unusual approach in Chapter 7.

Chapter 7

Illness as a Way of Life

Occasionally, a physician develops a relationship with a patient who is not only "sick all the time," but also worried about being sick all the time. No matter how many negative tests or normal examinations this patient has, the obsession that he or she has some medical disease continues. Being ill has become a way of life that the patient refuses to abandon. A person who behaves in this way is called a hypochondriac.

It is important to make clear that hypochondriacs do not lie about their symptoms. They do have pains, they do experience chronic fatigue, unrefreshing sleep, impaired memory, anxiety, muscle pains, bloating, chest pain, stiffness, diarrhea, depression, tingling sensations in the skin, difficulty concentrating, dry eyes and mouth, or a number of other ordinary and extraordinary symptoms. What a hypochondriac does *not* have is the disease he or she insists, despite all medical evidence to the contrary, is producing these symptoms: fibromyalgia, chronic fatigue syndrome, hypoglycemia or any of a dozen so called diseases whose symptoms are fully catalogued these days on the Internet.

Of all the patients I have seen with puzzling symptoms, hypochondriacs, as a group, are the most difficult and the most frustrating to try to help. It is as though they are determined to reject all help even before it is offered. They refuse to keep a diary of their symptoms to see if some toxic substance is causing them. They refuse to consider that a toxic relationship or social situation may produce their symptoms. They often reject, out of hand, the idea that stress can cause bodily symptoms. Suggesting that they see a psychologist or psychiatrist prompts a defensive reaction. Most patients in this group of disorders push their family and friends to the limit. Their complaints control the lives of those closest to them and they often end up separated from those who loved them the most.

There are many medical theories to explain hypochondria but no general agreement on its etiology, or cause. My own sense is that no single cause produces the obsessions with being ill. I have had very little success in my years of practice getting these patients to give up their obsessions by appealing to their conscious minds. If you are the family member of a hypochondriac, you will very likely not be able to "talk" this person out of his or her belief in the disease either.

Here is what Drs. Vladan Starcevic and Don R. Lipsitt said in their comprehensive review ("Hypochondriasis: Modern Perspectives on an Ancient Malady," Oxford University Press, 2001): "Hypochondriasis remains controversial, despite its 2000 year history. Although it is considered a mental disorder, hypochondriasis is often regarded as a defense mechanism, a peculiar cognitive/perceptual style, a means of nonverbal communication, a response to stress, an abnormal illness behavior, a personality trait, a distinct personality disturbance, and as a part of other mental disorders. Disagreements about the etiology and pathogenesis of hypochondriasis go hand in hand with disagreements about its treatment."

I have sometimes imagined being able to address the hypochondriac's unconscious mind. If I could, I would explain to him or her that the obsession with illness very likely arises from one or more of the following origins:

1. You learned early that the sick role was an effective way to back people away from you.

You learned in childhood to manipulate the sympathy that illness generates for your own benefit. You learned you could skip school, avoid chores, stay home, and play, if you said you were sick. The habit stuck. Sickness became a way of life early for you and your symptoms became real. Your parents most likely reinforced this behavior.

2. You were abused physically, emotionally, or sexually as a young child.

You learned that injury or illness removed or even prevented further abuse in the short run. You learned the power that sickness provided you. The pattern of behavior stuck. Illness became a maladaptive way of life long after the abuse stopped.

3. You were raised by health-obsessive parents who rushed you to the doctor at every bobble of your health – the slightest cough, the slightest fever, or even the hint of a pain.

It is no wonder your conscious mind thinks a medical disease lurks behind every symptom. You were taught to think and behave in this anxious way. Illness became your way of life.

4. You fell into a habit of refusing help from doctors and discovered that fooling doctors had a certain thrill.

When you did see a doctor, whatever he prescribed made you worse. If you had an operation, you got terrible complications. No pain pills worked and most made you feel sick. If you are in this group, you changed doctors frequently or you left the physician as soon as you defeated his efforts to help you. One of your hidden goals in life is to defeat experts. Maybe some of the experts resemble one or both of your parents, and you are getting back at them. Your conscious mind does not know that the best way to defeat the medical world is to stay healthy.

If I could speak in this way to the hypochondriac's unconscious mind, I would encourage him or her to consider which of these narratives fits best. Even though the conscious mind has rejected all of these explanations, I would speak in the hope that the unconscious mind would slowly but surely prompt the hypochondriac to see the cause of his or her obsessions with being ill.

Here are a few stories about patients of mine who had multiple symptoms. No matter what their doctor did or said, they never gave up the conviction that their symptoms were caused by a hidden medical disease, yet to be diagnosed. While all of these stories are about female patients, the literature on hypochondria includes many cases of male patients, too.

+   +   +

Miss Cootsie and Little Cootsie

Miss Cootsie lived on the top floor of her large Victorian mansion. From this perch, she had a commanding view of the street outside her home. She was in her eighties. Her daughter, Little Cootsie, lived in an adjoining bedroom with a connecting bathroom, which had been converted into a makeshift kitchen. Little Cootsie, now in her sixties and never married, had devoted her life to caring for her mother.

The entire first floor of the house had been closed off for years. All of the furniture was draped with old graying cloths.

The year was 1961. I was new to town and the youngest member of the medical group, so I was assigned the duty of making house calls to all the shut-ins, or "invalids," as they were called in those days. That's how I met Miss Cootsie. I didn't know it at the time, but Miss Cootsie had outlived four doctors before me. When I first saw her, I thought I was meeting Queen Victoria in person. The resemblance was striking, but there was one big difference. Miss Cootsie had the largest goiter in her neck that I had ever seen. It hung there, like two large oranges, dangling over the upper part of her chest, pulsating with each heart beat. I could not take my eyes off of it. Miss Cootsie had refused surgery for the goiter time after time and she quickly told me that.

As a newly trained endocrinologist, one especially trained in thyroid diseases, I could not believe what had just fallen into my hands. Everybody in town knew Miss Cootsie and her goiter. I just could not wait to shrink that goiter with thyroid hormone and make my reputation. The hormone would cut off the stimulus to grow, and the goiter would shrink back to normal size, or so I thought. I prescribed a small dose of thyroid hormone and gloated in my potential rise to fame.

In about two weeks, I got a call from Little Cootsie in the middle of the night. Miss Cootsie had gone stark raving mad and was running around the yard in her underwear. Little Cootsie said to come quickly. By the time I arrived, the sheriff had cornered Miss Cootsie and urged her into his car.

At the hospital, I found that Miss Cootsie had extreme hyperthyroidism. Little Cootsie told me that she thought her mother had taken the whole bottle of thyroid hormone and thus intoxicated herself into hyperthyroidism. Miss Cootsie proceeded to run a very toxic and dangerous course over the next several weeks in the hospital, progressing from acute heart failure, to pneumonia, then to a fulminate peeling skin rash from a reaction to penicillin. I finally got her back home and back to her front window view of the world. On my future house calls I listened only for the most dangerous symptoms and left Miss Cootsie alone. I learned quickly that some patients do not want to be cured and whoever tries to effect a cure does so at their own peril.

Comment:

Miss Cootsie was my first encounter as a physician with homebound shut-ins. I did not understand that she would resist any improvement in health I suggested. Her life and her daughter's were arranged around the idea of her illness. Her daughter suspected her mother had sabotaged her medications yet took no preventive measures to see that this would not occur. A hypochondriac sometimes secures an enabler.

+   +   +

Adelaine's headaches and her dutiful daughter

Adelaine was admitted to the psychiatric unit for deep depression and was scheduled for electric shock treatment. I was asked to evaluate her medical condition. A day before the treatment, she told me that she had moved to town a few months previously, following the death of her husband, and because her daughter had urged her to move to town to be nearby. Her daughter had helped her mother find a job at one of the department stores.

One night, shortly after moving to town, Adelaine slipped on the wet floor in her kitchen and fell. As she fell, she hit her head on the wooden island in her kitchen and knocked herself unconscious. When she came to, she reached out, found the phone, and called her daughter. She told her daughter of the fall and that her head hurt severely. The daughter rushed over and took her mother to the emergency room. Imaging studies and tests were normal and she was released.

Every few nights after her fall in the kitchen, Adelaine developed intense headaches. Each time this occurred, she called her daughter. Each time, the daughter rushed to the side of her mother. For the first several times, she took her mother back to the emergency room. Each time, she was released. Thereafter, when Adelaine called with a headache, the daughter would still rush to Adelaine's house and sit with her mother to provide comfort. This had become a regular pattern.

In addition to the recurring headaches, Adelaine became more and more depressed during this time. She felt alone in a new city, with no husband, in a new job, and now with severe headaches with no relief in sight. After I related this story to the psychiatrist who had admitted her, he decided to cancel the shock treatments and try medications for a while. Adelaine was discharged on an antidepressant drug.

I met with Adelaine's daughter just before Adelaine was discharged. It was obvious she was at wit's end about what to do with her mother. Hearing the story, I thought it plausible that Adelaine's headaches had become a conditioned response. In other words, the solicitous reactions of the daughter rushing to the mother had somehow reinforced the headaches.

I suggested to the daughter a different approach. The next time her mother phoned her to report a headache, she was to say to her mother, "Oh, Mother, I am so sorry you are hurting. I do not want to add worry to your headaches. I want to see you when you feel better and we can visit and talk. I hope you feel better soon." She was then to hang up and not go to her mother's house.

I also requested that she not go to her mother's home unless her mother called and did not mention her headache. In other words, the daughter was to ignore headache signals and reward healthy signals. I also advised her never to inquire about headaches in the future. After her daughter had followed this approach for a few weeks, Adelaine's headaches did not return and her depression lifted on the antidepressant medication.

Comment:

There is an old dictum in behavior modification that any negative behavior ignored will be extinguished. In other words, if you pay no attention to an undesirable behavior long enough, then the behavior will go away. This is no cure-all or panacea, and it often fails, as old dicta often do. However, it is worth a try. It seemed to work with Adelaine and her daughter, in combination with the antidepressant drug.

+   +   +

A woman with seizures

I once saw a woman in her sixties, Mrs. Quint, whose family believed she was pretending to suffer epileptic seizures in order to get their attention. They told me that when a "seizure" occurred, Mrs. Quint would scream out, flail her arms, and her body would jerk up and down. Sometimes she would spin in circles. She would wake suddenly and appear to have no memory of the attack. Each time she had one of these spells, the whole Quint family would gather at her home to be sure she was "alright."

The seizure workup I ordered for Mrs. Quint was negative, and she had no electroencephalographic (EEG) pattern of a seizure disorder. The CT scan of her head was normal, as was her neurological exam. The evidence was clear both from the negative workup and the bizarre description of her seizures that she had feigned the epileptic attacks. Her family's response only reinforced the behavior.

A psychiatrist and I met with all of the grown Quint children. We presented them with the results of my tests and examination and suggested that the next time their mother had a "seizure," they should ignore it. Of course, the child who was present when the fit occurred should make sure she did not injure herself, but otherwise the child should back off and watch. The other children should not be called to the house. They were not doing anything anyway when they ran to her side. They all agreed to try the plan.

Mrs. Quint's oldest daughter called the psychiatrist for a follow up a few weeks later. She reported that her mother had had a seizure as soon as they got home from their appointment with us. When no one paid any attention, Mrs. Quint started sliding across the floor and spinning in circles on the floor trying to trip her daughter with her feet. When her daughter moved across the room, Mrs. Quint slid in the same direction, still jerking on the floor.

The psychiatrist reinforced our suggestion to ignore the seizures and added that any family members present, when one occurred, should actually step over Mrs. Quint when she had seizures. The seizure-like episodes continued for another two months, dwindled in frequency, and then stopped.

Comment:

When there is a specific illness behavior, then having the family ignore the behavior may work. When the illness behavior is diffuse and the symptoms widespread in different parts of the body, then ignoring the illness becomes impossible.

Dr. Marc Feldman (Author of *Playing Sick*) would say that Mrs.Quint actually has a factitious disorder (not hypochondriasis) since she is feigning her illness (See Chapter 8 for clarification.). I include her story in this chapter because of the family dynamics.

+   +   +

Mrs. Oliver Townwell's life in a wheelchair

Here is one more story, this time not from my own but from a colleague's practice. Mrs. Townwell (again not her real name) was the wife of a prominent insurance broker in a small town in Mississippi. Shortly after the birth of her second child, Mrs. Townwell developed weakness in her legs. She was seen by many doctors, but no one could identify the cause for the muscle weakness. In a few years, she could not stand without assistance and was soon confined to a wheelchair.

Her two daughters married and had children. Both lived in

houses down the street from their parents. Even though Mrs. Townwell lived with Mr. Townwell throughout their marriage, their daughters had, since leaving home, always rotated spending nights with their partially paralyzed mother.

Twenty-three years after Mrs. Townwell was confined to a wheelchair, Mr. Townwell dropped dead in his office. At the funeral, Mrs. Townwell got up from her wheelchair and walked defiantly to the graveside. She never used the wheelchair again. She never explained or discussed her weakness. However, it was eventually learned that Mr. Townwell had begun a love affair with his secretary when Mrs. Townwell was pregnant with their second child, and before she developed weakness in her legs. The secret apparently explained her weakness and her need for perpetual help while he lived.

Comment:

In his studies of families, Dr. Murray Bowen observed that chronic illness in a spouse will stabilize and sustain a marriage (*Family Therapy in Clinical Practice*, New York, NY: Aronson, 1978). I doubt that Mrs. Townwell ever read or heard of Dr. Bowen, but her story verifies his observations. By her paralysis, Mrs. Townwell controlled both the continuation of her marriage and the devotion of her two daughters.

Each of the cases I have related here — Miss Cootie, Adelaine, Mrs. Quint, and Mrs. Townwell — involved patients whose whole illness controlled and was reinforced by family members. If you recognize a family member in these stories, you may benefit from consulting Dr. Marc Feldman's *Playing Sick*. (New York: Brunner-Rutledge, 2004). Dr. Feldman is an authority on patients who have multiple symptoms and an obsession about having a medical disease. Along with his many other helpful suggestions, he provides the following list of suggestions to people who are worried about having a serious medical disease despite being assured by their physicians, after comprehensive medical examinations, that they do not have a medical disease. My experience is that, while it is very difficult to get a hypochondriac to give up his or her obsession, educating family members and encouraging them not to cater to the obsessions sometimes does lead to healthier situations. Take a look at the list, and consider how you might help "your hypochondriac" put these techniques into practice.

1. Keeping a journal describing symptoms or events that led to your anxiety or panic attacks, or episodes of illness worry, should allow one to see a closer link between one's symptoms and external events.

2. Trying to restrict or put a time limit on one's Internet medical research, reading of medical books, or self-checking behaviors, as they tend to increase illness worries.

3. Maintaining a healthy lifestyle, including a good night's sleep, well-balanced diet, and a positive outlook. A good tip is to follow the PEAS tool sometimes used to combat depression: Pleasure, Exercise, Achievement and Socializing — try to add an aspect of each to daily activities.

4. Practicing relaxation techniques, such as breathing, meditation, or other methods may help to decrease anxiety and the effects of stress.

5. Trying to interrupt one's worries with activities that will fully engage one's attention and shift it away from illness; for example, hobbies, word or number games, exercise or walking, talking with a humorous friend, or recalling happy memories.

6. Thinking about alternative explanations for one's physical sensations that might include stress or normal bodily changes.

7. Breaking one's habits of worrying, one step at a time.

Additional Suggestions:

Here are some additional suggestions I make to families for coping with hypochondriacs.

First, try to help him or her avoid unnecessary surgery and unnecessary emergency room visits. Get second opinions for all suggested elective procedures.

Second, ensure he or she gets regular checkups by a single general physician. The time interval between visits becomes very important. Some of these patients need to be seen every week or two. Some can be seen every month or two.

Third, all specialist consultations should be ordered ideally only by this one general physician. Specialist reports should go in writing only to the primary care physician, and if possible, consultants should not discuss their findings with the patient. They are only consultants to the primary physician. This will take a special arrangement between the specialist and the primary physician. Having many doctors only fuels the patient's worries about hidden disease. One doctor, if possible, should do all of the talking with the patient. These limitations take some time and effort to orchestrate but they are worth it in the long run. Limiting the advice to one physician is worth the effort.

Fourth, be sure that good medical care is provided regularly so that no treatable medical disease is overlooked. Don't forget that these patients, like all humans, will eventually get a disease.

Fifth, all drugs should be kept to a minimum and prescribed only by the single generalist physician.

During the twelve year period that I studied patients with puzzling symptoms I saw twenty-one patients whom I considered to be hypochondriacs; that is, people for whom illness had become a way of life. None had any detectable medical disease. None were depressed. All carried one or more diagnoses of nonexistent diseases, and all took several medications a day. The average number of symptoms was over fifteen. I was able to persuade only two of these twenty-one patients to stop the medications and to drop the false diagnoses.

As I gained experience with this group of patients, I learned to ask two very revealing questions. The first is: "When were you last in robust good health?" I will never forget one woman, in her fifties, who said, "I have never been well a day in my life. The day I was born, the obstetrician dropped me on the delivery room floor. My mother told me I was never well after that."

The second question is: "If you suddenly got well, were free of all of your symptoms, and could do anything you wanted to do, what would you do differently?" Hypochondriacs are confused, even bewildered, by this question. Often their response is just a blank look. Illness is the only way of life that seems viable. Good health does not appear, even theoretically, to be an option.

In my practice, the only rule I found truly helpful with patients who reject all objective offers of help is the ancient rule, known to all physicians:

Primum non nocere

(First, do no harm.)

It takes very special physicians to care for these patients and avoid unnecessary drugs and surgery. You are lucky if you can find one.

Chapter 8

Self Infliction and Feigned Illnesses:
The Most Puzzling Symptoms

In the previous chapters I have shared with you stories about patients whose puzzling symptoms are misdiagnosed and mistreated. I have stressed that when a full medical workup by your physician (medical exam, laboratory work, imaging studies, and careful history review) does not reveal a medical disease as the cause of your symptoms, it is important for you to keep a careful diary of your symptoms, consider what substances you may be exposed to or ingesting, and examine your living conditions, work situation, and personal relationships for stress which may produce your symptoms. I have repeated that you must ask yourself two important questions as you make entries in your diary:

What am I doing in my life that I should not be doing?
What am I not doing in my life that I should be doing?

This advice is all predicated on my acceptance of your symptoms as real and my confident belief that causes for real symptoms can be discovered through careful detective work and diary keeping.

There is an entirely different set of puzzling symptoms that physicians sometimes encounter. In this chapter, I will take a closer look at these situations for the sake of contrast with the symptoms you are very likely experiencing. No diary keeping will help patients with symptoms of the kind this chapter concerns.

The most puzzling symptoms that a physician encounters are those that are self-inflicted or feigned. "Self Harm" is the newly suggested term for disorders in this group of patients. Marc

Feldman in his encyclopedic book *Playing Sick* (New York, NY: Brunner-Rutledge, 2004), suggests four separable disorders: Munchausen Syndrome, Munchausen by Proxy, Malingering, and Factitious Disorder. The common feature of these disorders is that these patients deliberately inflict harm or injury on themselves, feign symptoms, and then deny the injury is self-inflicted. People with Munchausen by Proxy inflict harm on another person, usually a child, to produce illness and disease.

Munchausen Syndrome was named for a real Baron von Munchausen, an eighteenth-century German aristocrat. He had a reputation for telling tall tales, and stories about his fantastical adventures were circulated in the nineteenth century. Patients with Munchausen Syndrome move from town to town telling incredible stories about their made-up illnesses. They also inflict real harm on themselves through elaborate means, such as injecting feces into themselves, taking anticoagulants, bleeding themselves, injecting insulin, or feigning serious neurological disorders. The list of injuries goes on and on. The psychological gain here is attention and acceptance that cannot be obtained by normal human social interaction. This syndrome is best considered to be a psychiatric disorder.

Munchausen by Proxy is defined as someone inflicting injury on another person to produce a disease. Most often this is a mother inflicting disease on one of her children. This is a crime, but dispute exists about whether it is also a psychiatric disorder. Either way, it should always be reported to the police.

Malingering is conscious infliction or feigning of an illness for drugs, or monetary or other tangible gain. This often co-exists with a personality disorder, such as a borderline or antisocial personality.

Factitious disorders are defined as self-inflicted or feigned illnesses. These conditions differ from Munchausen Syndrome in that these patients tend to stay in one place and can be employed and to some extent live productive lives. True Munchausen patients are completely consumed by the sham and lead lives devoted to being in hospitals, getting operated on surgically, moving from town to town, and tricking doctors with elaborate schemes of deception. The gain is often the excitement of fooling experts, even at the peril of their lives.

For a long time these problems were thought to be rare. Recent surveys, however, according to Marc Feldman, reveal that 9.3 percent of tertiary care-level patients have factitious disorders and that 1.3 percent of outpatients have the disorder (personal communication). Munchausen and factitious disorder patients find a wide variety of methods for inflicting self-harm, as you will see in the following stories.

+   +   +

A nurse with large bruises

Miss V.N., a nursing instructor, was twenty-eight years old. She came to see me about large deep purple bruises over her abdomen, arms, and thighs. She taught at a nursing school in a community college in an adjoining town.

As I did the initial physical examination, she often interjected dramatic statements about her previous health. For example, as I examined her left eye, she said, "Oh, I had a time with that eye. When I was with my mother and father in the jungles of Indonesia on a mission trip, I cut my eye with a butcher knife. The eye fluid ran all over my face."

Taken back, I asked how she now had a normal eye. She told me that there had been an excellent surgeon in the mission hospital and that he sewed the eye up immediately. I knew at once that this was impossible, and remained alert to possible fabrication for the remainder of the examination.

With almost every organ I examined, Miss V.N. related some

serious illness she had had as a child and detailed as well a complete recovery. Her heart had escaped serious mitral valve damage from rheumatic fever. Her lungs had healed following a deep fungus infection. She had had parasites in her liver, now gone. She had had cholera and typhoid fever and an endless series of serious illnesses. She had recovered from each with no residual.

I commented how remarkable it was that she appeared to be in such excellent health. She smiled broadly and said nothing.

Studies of her clotting system showed prolonged clotting times. The prolonged time for her blood to clot returned to normal when protamine was added to her blood in the laboratory. Protamine reverses the effects of the drug heparin, so these findings could only be explained by injected heparin, a strong anticoagulant. Heparin, which thins the blood and often results in bruising, explained Miss V.N.'s puzzling symptoms.

I asked for a psychiatric consultation. Together the psychiatrist and I confronted Miss V.N. about the heparin injections. She vehemently denied injecting herself.

The psychiatrist and I had worked together on a number of patients so we agreed to try to help Miss V.N. The year was 1977, long before Dr. Feldman and others more clearly defined these disorders and described methods for treating these patients. Both of us knew at the time, however, that most patients with self-inflicted wounds or diseases will not return for care. Once the cause of the injury is discovered, they move on to other physicians. We were hopeful of gaining some understanding of the causes of such aberrant behavior.

A few weeks later I was called to the emergency room where I found Miss V.N. lying on a bed, smiling and talking to a nurse. She had a large abscess deep in the muscle of her left upper arm. Cultures later revealed staphylococcus. She told me that she had been letting her nursing students practice injections on her and she thought one must have broken sterile technique. I stepped out in the hallway and called the head of the nursing school where she taught. She told me that practice injections were forbidden. I confronted Miss V.N. with this information. She insisted she was telling the truth.

We admitted Miss V.N. to the short stay unit since the abscess drainage would require a deep incision and drainage. On the following day, when I entered her room, I found Miss V.N. letting blood run out of her IV tubing into the trash can. She was bleeding herself. There was a large amount of blood in the can. Her hemoglobin level was very low.

I called the psychiatrist, and we arranged a commitment to the psychiatric unit. Short involuntary commitment was still possible in those days if patients posed harm to themselves or others. At this point I had reached the limits of my expertise. I told the psychiatrist and the patient that I would be resigning her care at discharge. I wrote her a letter asking her to get another physician within two weeks.

The psychiatrist told me he would continue seeing Miss V.N. because he thought he could help her. After she went home, he told me every few weeks that he was making progress and that she was gaining insight.

Then Miss V.N. disappeared. Six months later, I got a call from a physician in a city in Florida. He said Miss V.N. was in his office and told him that she had been under treatment by me for acute leukemia but that she was in remission. I told him the whole story and wished him well. I never heard from Miss V.N., nor about her, again.

Comment:

In the 1970s, most physicians saw disorders like Miss V.N.'s as not treatable, as I did. Most of us dismissed these patients from our practices. As I mentioned, Marc Feldman's *Playing Sick* gives an extensive review of these syndromes and modes of confronting and helping some of these patients. Families with members with these problems are urged to help these people seek long-term psychiatric care.

Today, Miss V.N. would be labeled Munchausen Syndrome because she moved about and because she told very tall tales. Her case illustrates the extremes of lying and of inflicting self-harm that Munchausen patients will go to in an effort to secure medical attention and confuse physicians.

+ + +

A teenager with multiple abscesses of her legs

I was a medical resident when Lucie, a teenage girl, was admitted on multiple occasions for extensive deep abscesses in her thighs and calves. Over several years, she lost much of the muscle tissue of her calves, and her skin was tightly bound to the underlying bones of her legs. She could walk only with crutches. The disfigurement was extreme and contrasted sharply with the beauty of Lucie's face and upper body.

It was found during one of her admissions that she was injecting herself with an insecticide. No one had been able to convince her to stop nor had repeated confinements to the psychiatric unit been of any help.

Comment:

The number and kinds of substances that are self-injected by patients with these disorders are nearly limitless. These types of cases can go undetected for long periods until some person suspects self-harm and uncovers the real cause. Treatment often fails because many of these patients disappear or move on to other physicians. Lucie would be classified as having a factitious disorder. These patients seek attention, warm human contact, and caring attention, and may inflict serious and lasting harm on themselves in the effort to achieve these ends. Some of these patients, if carefully approached by a team of physicians, nurses, and psychiatrists, can be helped. There are now reports of patients in remission for long periods of time. You can read extensive reports of such treatments in Feldman's *Playing Sick.*

+   +   +

A woman with bruises and a low blood sugar

When I was a medical resident, we admitted T.J., a woman in her late thirties, for seizures and multiple bruises of her skin. She was in good health otherwise. Laboratory tests initially showed a low blood sugar that returned to normal after a few hours. Tests for clotting showed low prothrombin activity in her blood. Prothrombin is an essential chemical for clotting of blood. Many diseases can cause a reduction in prothrombin. The combination of a low blood sugar and a clotting disorder provoked all sorts of strange speculations and guesses.

T.J.'s skin was bruised over much of her body. Each bruise was paired with another identical bruise. These are called butterfly bruises because they resemble small butterflies. No bruises were present on the skin of her back in the area between her shoulder blades. The appearance of the butterfly bruises and their absence in an area T.J. could not reach easily meant only one thing. She had pinched herself to produce the widespread bruising. The clotting defect and low prothrombin activity were later found to be due to ingestion of the anticoagulant Coumadin. When confronted with the other information, she also admitted to insulin injections to produce the low blood sugar.

Comment:

T.J.'s case illustrates the extremes that patients with self-inflicted symptoms will go to in order to present clinical puzzles. T.J.

was injecting insulin, taking Coumadin, and pinching herself to make bruises. She signed out against medical advice and was lost to follow-up. She would be classified as having a factitious disorder.

+ + +

Another kind of self-harm with a different motivation

Mrs. L.H. was in her late forties when I met her, and was admitted with renal colic (pain typical of passing a kidney stone). This was her fifth admission for renal colic.

I was asked to see her as a metabolic consultant to try to find out what kinds of kidney stones she was passing. Previous attempts to find fragments of stones in her urine had failed. All of her blood chemistries were normal, which ruled out most of the common causes for renal stones. All of her urine examinations contained large amounts of red blood cells, a finding typical with passing kidney stones.

When I entered the room, I was a bit surprised to find Mrs. L.H. sitting in a chair, especially since she was writhing in pain. I asked all the standard questions and did my physical examination. She had very poor dental hygiene with swollen gums and many cavities in her teeth. She asked repeatedly for more narcotics.

Straining her urine into the special container attached to the toilet yielded small brown fragments. When analyzed in the lab, the stones were found to be mostly xanthine. I had never heard of a xanthine stone. Just as we began to look in the literature to find out about xanthine stones, the nurse called me to the floor. She had just caught Mrs. L.H. kneeling by the toilet, picking her gums with pecan shells, and letting the blood and shells drip into the urine collection. When confronted, she denied doing this right in the face of the nurse who saw her do it.

Comment:

Unlike Miss V.N., Mrs. L.H. was not attempting to get attention but to satisfy her addiction to narcotics. Dr. Feldman would classify her as a malingerer because she was seeking a tangible, and not a psychological, reward. By the way, pecan shells will analyze as being high in xanthine-like compounds. Had the nurse not seen the self-inflicted bleeding, I can imagine lengthy grand rounds discussing xanthine kidney stones!

+ + +

Recurring fever with air under the skin

This case history was told over and over by residents at Vanderbilt Hospital many years ago. I recorded the story in two of my books–*Med School* and *Twentieth Century Men of Medicine: Personal Reflections*. The story is worth telling again because it illustrates how difficult it can be for a doctor to get an accurate history, and how strange that history may turn out to be. The story also illustrates how unusual an injected substance can be.

Sam, a young man in his twenties, was repeatedly admitted for a curious combination of high fever and air under the skin of his chest which spread down into both upper arms. This is called subcutaneous emphysema, which is a mixture of Greek and Latin for "air under the skin." The skin of people with this condition has a crunchy feel that is unmistakable for anything else. The condition is always rare and is usually produced by a rib fracture that tears the lung, allowing air to leak under the skin of the chest. There were no rib fractures in this patient.

The case was presented on several occasions over a year, at the weekly grand round conference. Many diagnostic suggestions of bizarre and unusual connections between his trachea or esophagus and the skin were explored. None were ever found. Some doctors suggested a new gas-forming bacterium was the cause. At each admission he was given antibiotics and the fever went away as did the air under the skin. Sam remained a medical diagnostic puzzle and a challenge until Dr. Rudolph Kampmeier, the master diagnostician, was finally called to see the young man.

Here is the history he obtained, one which no one previously had managed to extract from the young man: Sam lived in the country with his family. His father ran a gas station a short distance from their home. Every few nights, Sam's girlfriend walked over from her house, a few hundred yards away. They met in the back of the gas station and had sexual intercourse, but not the usual kind. The girl had persuaded Sam to let her pump him up with air from a football pump. She bit a small hole in his arm, inserted the needle of the pump, and pumped enough air to fill out the skin of his chest and back. She liked the crunchy feel of the air under his skin. Sam did not mind. On most occasions, nothing bad happened. However, whenever he developed fever, he knew he would receive treatment at the hospital and that he would get well. In addition to getting the true history, Kampmeier saw to it that Sam stopped the practice. He did not present again.

Comment:

This case shows the elaborate collusions that can go on between two consenting people. This case differs from the Munchausen by Proxy cases, where one person intentionally inflicts harm on another person and fully intends to produce abnormal findings and injury. Often in these cases, a mother does this surreptitiously to her child.

In this case, there was no intention to produce harm—quite the opposite. The intent was a desire to heighten sexual pleasure, but the bizarre means chosen proved unsanitary and dangerous. The infection Sam developed from time to time came from a dirty bicycle pump and from saliva contamination in the bite. There was collusion only to keep the truth from being known to the doctors, not to do harm.

Here are two additional cases where people harm themselves unintentionally, but do not attempt to deceive their doctors.

+ + +

An old woman with a low blood potassium level

I was asked to see Mrs. G.O. to evaluate her low blood potassium level. Mrs. G.O. was eighty years old and a grandmother to ten children. Low potassium levels can come from gastrointestinal loss (either through vomiting or diarrhea) or from excretion of excess potassium in the urine. If the potassium level in the urine is very low, it means the loss is from the GI tract or from previous kidney excretion. Finding that Mrs. G.O.'s urine potassium level was very low suggested that she was doing one of three things–secretly vomiting, taking diuretics and not admitting it, or using large amounts of laxatives secretly. In general, the older the patient, the more likely it will be laxative abuse.

There is a way of questioning in these situations that increases the likelihood of a truthful answer. Most people who are secretly vomiting, sneaking diuretics, or abusing laxatives will not want to admit it. Coming at these questions indirectly is the best strategy to get to the truth. If I say, "Are you taking large amounts of laxative?" then I will likely get a denial. In fact, the intern had already got a denial of excessive laxative use from Mrs. G.O. when he put the question directly.

A friend of mine had invented what he called the "ubiquity question." It is useful whenever you are seeking information that could be embarrassing. In this situation with Mrs. G.O., I said, "Mrs. O., a lot of patients I see take laxatives every day. Some I know take a bottle of Milk of Magnesia daily. Some have to take four or five bottles a day. How many do you take?"

She quickly answered, "Oh, I only take two bottles a day."

The "ubiquity question" permits a wide range of answers, and it permits, even sanctions, almost any behavior. In self-inflicting situations, it sometimes is the best way to try to get a truthful answer.

Comment:

Laxative and enema abuse are common in old people. Constipation seems to be ever present, and it is possible that some sort of pleasure is produced by the forceful bowel movement induced by laxatives or enemas. I do know it is a difficult problem, and many patients continue to take excessive amounts of laxative even when admonished not to do so. Low potassium levels can be dangerous and trigger abnormal heart rhythms. In severe potassium depletion, muscle weakness can be extreme with loss of ability to walk, as you will see in the case that follows.

Families with older members who are unusually weak should be alert to laxative abuse. The motivation for these patients is not attention or reward. These patients are quite the opposite from the self-dramatizing Munchausen Syndrome type. People with laxative abuse hide and deny the problem. Many of them believe it improves their health and resist the idea that they are harming themselves.

+   +   +

A bizarre habit still seen in the rural South

Miss B.N. was a nineteen-year-old unmarried sharecropper who was pregnant for the third time. She was referred to the medical center because she was partially paralyzed and had a very low blood potassium level. In addition she was having periodic bursts of very fast heartbeats (ventricular tachycardia).

Her urine potassium was low, suggesting a gastrointestinal loss of potassium. She denied vomiting or diarrhea or laxative abuse. She also denied previous use of diuretics. She said every time she got pregnant, she developed the severe weakness and the rapid heartbeat. The first two pregnancies ended in the second trimester with spontaneous miscarriages. This was the first time she had sought medical care with her pregnancy.

Initial lab work did not reveal the cause of Miss B.N.'s symptoms.

It was only when her aunt visited her that we discovered the source of her potassium loss. The aunt told us that it was common in that area for pregnant girls to eat clay. The clay had a sweet taste and pregnancy brought out a craving for the taste of the clay. The aunt wondered if there might be a connection between eating clay and her niece's condition.

The clay was gray-colored and came from a special bank near a river. When we explored this further with Miss B.N., she admitted eating nearly a pint of clay a day. "Pica," or the eating of non-nutritive substances, was so widespread in the area that no one (except Miss B.N.'s aunt) had considered it possibly to be unhealthy or dangerous.

After repletion with large amounts of oral and intravenous potassium, Miss B.N. regained her full strength and her rapid heartbeat stopped. She went on to a full-term normal pregnancy and delivery.

Comment:

In this case again, intake of a substance accounts for the unusual symptoms. Here, the patient did not hide the substance from the doctor, but did not report it in her history because it was such common practice to consume it when pregnant. It took an astute observer, like the aunt, to make the connection between the clay eating and the illness. The clay Miss B.N. ate was mostly diatomaceous earth. It is formed from small diatoms that floated in the prehistoric oceans and later settled into clay banks.

When we tested it in the laboratory, the clay was able to bind and trap large amounts of potassium. Potassium was trapped by the clay in the gastrointestinal tract and defecated, robbing Miss B.N. of an important bodily substance.

Clay eating is still common in many areas of the rural south. It was very common among slaves, and often led to death. The association with potassium loss, of course, was unknown, but the condition was known as *Cachexia Africanus* and was reported in the medical literature in the mid 1800s.

For those of you with puzzling symptoms, I want to emphasize that self-inflicted conditions are not the main thrust of this book. My primary concern is with puzzling symptoms whose cause is most often exposure to a substance or a situational stress which can be proved to cause the symptom. However, no book on puzzling symptoms could be complete without including these cases of self-harm, not only because they are more widespread than formerly believed, as reported by Dr. Feldman, but also because they often become dangerous and life-threatening conditions. My hope is that the cases reported here will alert families who suspect their relative has a self-inflicted condition to seek professional help and to recognize the danger of the situation.

Chapter 9

Alcoholism: The Hidden Disease

Of all diseases, there is one diagnosis that is most often missed or overlooked in American medicine. It can produce almost any symptom, so you need to consider carefully if you or a member of your family could be a victim.

The disease is very common, affecting over seventeen million Americans and causing pain and anguish to over eighty million family members. It is invariably fatal unless identified and managed. It is a progressive disease, getting worse with every passing year. It cannot be cured but it can be treated and controlled. Sadly, the disease is often denied by its victims even at the point of death.

The disease is alcohol addiction. Its victims are chronic alcoholics.

Alcohol abuse is even more common, accounting for a large percentage of serious automobile injuries and death. Both alcohol addiction and alcohol abuse can be silent and missed by physicians and families for long periods of time. Some patients will deny alcohol abuse or addiction even when they are on their dying beds.

Both abuse and addiction are extremely tricky diagnoses to make. Alcoholism has been misunderstood by many health professionals, including myself. Until very recently, I had a large misrepresentation of what I thought alcohol addiction was. I had the misconception that chronic alcoholism was always *secondary* to some other condition. For example, I thought excessive drinking was in response to grief or depression, or to some painful memories of childhood, or a painful situation at work or in marriage. In other words I thought it was always a *secondary* disease. That is not the case for most alcoholics.

Alcohol addiction is a *primary* disease. That means it is a disease all to itself. It can and does exist alone, with no other associated state. Of course people sometimes drink heavily in response to acute situations. And certainly depression, anxiety, painful memories, and stressful situations do occur in the lives of alcoholics but they are not necessary conditions. Alcoholics are addicted to alcohol even in the complete absence of any co-existing conditions. As one recovering alcoholic told me, "Hell, I'll drink because the sun is shining outside." There does not have to be a reason to drink when one is an alcoholic. Craving alcohol is the sole drive and no amount of drinking will quench it. Abstinence is the only healthy course.

Here is the way alcohol addiction appears to work. First, the alcoholic has an inherited genetic predisposition to becoming addicted to alcohol. There is no way currently to test for the presence or absence of this gene. If a close relative (grandparent, parent, sibling, aunt, or uncle) is an alcoholic, then you are at risk for becoming an alcoholic. This does not mean you have the gene but you are at risk for having the gene. There is no way currently to predict exactly who will get the gene.

Without the genetic makeup, conventional wisdom says you are not at risk for becoming an alcohol addict. However, you still could be an alcohol abuser – more on alcohol abuse later.

If you do have the genetic predisposition, here is how alcohol addiction arises. You, or anyone with the genetic makeup, begins drinking alcoholic beverages. At first and in the early stages of alcoholism, this is done purely for the enhanced feelings of elation or euphoria. This period of drinking, only for the euphoric effect, is highly variable in length. It can run for many years. After a while, the brain no longer responds just to euphoria but it demands more alcohol and it does this by creating an intense craving. This intense craving increases until it completely controls the life of the alcoholic. Its intensity is akin to running out of breath twenty feet under water. The feeling of needing air and the drive to get to the surface for air are similar to the alcoholic's craving for alcohol. The craving is insatiable. Eventually, no amount of alcohol will quench it. The fruitless search to satisfy the craving begins the downward spiral toward death and arrests, family turmoil, loss of job, and divorce.

This craving can start with the first drink or it can occur many years after drinking begins. As the craving increases, so does the amount of alcohol consumed. No amount will eliminate the craving and slowly but surely the alcoholic is on the pathway to death. Alcoholism, unless controlled, is always a fatal disease. The liver becomes hardened and cirrhotic, the veins in the esophagus enlarge and rupture, leading often to fatal hemorrhages. The abdomen swells with collected fluid. The brain and nerves are damaged leading to gait and mental aberrations and dementia. The heart can fail. All of these changes progress to death. The only way out is for the alcoholic is to admit him or herself into treatment and learn to live with complete abstinence from alcohol.

There is one major factor that prevents the alcoholic from recognizing his or her problem. It is called denial – denial that is so real and so intense that reality is obliterated. My colleagues who specialize in treating alcoholics tell me stories of patients who completely denied drinking even as they vomited blood from their dilated esophageal veins. Unless the denial is overcome, the alcoholic will die from the toxic effects of alcohol. Again, for emphasis, alcoholism is a fatal progressive disease. I had one patient deny excessive drinking as he lay dying from liver failure from his alcoholic cirrhosis. Denial is powerful and it is real.

I doubt if many of you are who are reading this are admitted alcoholics. If you are then please seek intensive help which is available in many forms.

If you don't know if you are an alcoholic, then please take the MAST test in Appendix II. Be honest. You are searching for the causes of your symptoms. If you score high on the test, seek help. You might turn to your spouse or your companion or your family members. Ask them what they think of your drinking. Listen and accept their help and advice. Whatever you do, seek professional help.

The first step is to admit that alcohol has control of your life. Once you admit that, there are all sorts of help available to help keep you sober.

In addition to taking the MAST test, review the listed symptoms below. Most of these symptoms come from the toxic effects of alcohol. If you have one or more of any of these symptoms, you should consult your doctor for professional help: weakness, dizziness, substernal pain after eating (due to esophageal regurgitation), abdominal pain, unexplained panic attacks, swelling of the abdomen or increased belt size, inability to get an erection, male breast growth, sleep pattern disturbances, blood in the stool, and vomiting blood. Check the skin over your chest for tiny red spider angiomas and check for swelling of your ankles. Have you lost sensation in your feet or do your feet or hands tingle? None of these symptoms or physical findings is specific for alcoholism or alcohol abuse; however, all should be investigated medically.

If you are an alcoholic, you will not recall or admit to periods of mental blackouts. Ask your friends or relatives if you have had periods of mental blackouts. These events are highly suggestive of alcoholism.

Alcohol abuse can occur in non-alcoholics. The definition of alcohol abuse is highly variable from one person to another. If you, as a man, are drinking more than 100 drinks a month or as a woman, more than 80 drinks a month, then you are abusing alcohol. Just because you drink wine or beer, do not believe that you are escaping the toxic effects of alcohol. Here are the rough equivalents: A glass of wine equals twelve ounces of beer equals one shot of whiskey.

If you are a family member of an alcoholic, there are also all kinds of help available to you. Begin by seeking out an Al-Anon chapter and try attending at least three meetings. Talk to your physician or counselor for help. Read *Dying for a Drink* by Anderson Spickard, Jr., M.D. and Barbara R. Thompson (Nashville, TN: W Publishing Company, Thomas Nelson, 2005). This book explains the disease and gives solid advice to families on how to deal with a loved one's denial. Breaking through the denial is the first helpful step. You did not cause the problem, you cannot control the drinking, and you cannot cure the problem. You can, however, contribute to the problem by enabling the person to remain an alcoholic. Learn how you enable and how you can stop enabling the drinking. Educating yourself about alcoholism may help you learn the warning signs and alert you to your own genetic predisposition for this disease.

You may be the alcoholic's only hope. Seek professional help and guidance to assist you and your family in penetrating the denial of your alcoholic.

Chapter 10

Some Concluding Thoughts and Advice

The more I think about the diagnostic process, the more I now see that most of the marvelous new technology available to us today is visual. It is aimed at seeing disease. We have ultrasound for nearly every organ. We can look inside the small arteries of the heart. With the MRI we can see details of the brain and spinal cord or inside joints. We can outline nearly every organ and see very small tumors. With arteriography, we can detect narrowed vessels. All of our blood tests are visual in one way or another. We are in the age and era of medical visualization.

In one regrettable sense, medicine is on the verge of saying, "If we cannot see it, it does not exist."

However, diseases and dysfunctions often cannot be seen. Most of the patient examples in this book were heard and not seen. Medicine's over-reliance on seeing has led to a decline in physicians listening. The most frequent complaint I hear from patients is that they do not feel listened to by their physicians. While feeling listened to is important and even vital for human relationships, I am more concerned about the fact that listening is an essential diagnostic tool for many symptoms. In Chapter 1, I wrote about diseases that can be confirmed by testing. I also wrote about diseases that cannot be confirmed by testing. I spoke of the latter type of disease as characterized by templates or patterns or syndromes. All of these pattern-type diseases must be teased out mainly by talking and listening.

It is not enough to recognize a pattern of disease. It is not enough to say someone has spastic colon or a spastic bladder or tension headaches or a sore back or indigestion or constipation. The doctor and the patient must discover what about the patient and his or her life is causing the "pattern disease."

I suggested in Chapters 3, 4, and 5 that there are two very broad categories of causes:

1. Toxic social or personal encounters causing stress.
2. Toxic substances you are ingesting or inhaling, or that are making contact with your skin.

All of these causes of illness require that you pay close attention to the details of your life in order to discover what is uniquely offensive to you and your body and mind and spirit. Not only your doctor, but you, must become a better listener.

Despite the fact that enormous technical progress has been made in medical testing and treatment since I first began to practice medicine in the 1950s, one discouraging truth about tending to human health remains unchanged: If you are poor and uneducated and lack access to adequate medical care, you are far more likely to experience health-related pain and suffering. A fair amount of research has gone into exploring the relationship between socioeconomic status and health, and it supports what common sense tell us: People who begin life in a healthy environment, who are taught good health habits from the start, who keep informed about how diet, and exercise, and environment affect one's health, and who can afford good medical care usually live longer and have healthier lives. There is also good evidence that the most important socioeconomic factors influencing health are years of formal education and literacy. From education comes the ability to learn what is and is not good for you. In addition, there is nothing more stressful than being illiterate and poor in an affluent and literate society. None of the methods I've offered in this book to help you understand your puzzling symptoms will help you if you are significantly handicapped by socioeconomic factors beyond your control. This is a sad and humbling truth that doctors learn again and again over a lifetime of practice.

When I decided to write this book, I knew that I would be addressing a fairly select group of readers. Many of you, for one reason or another — a persistent tingling, an undiagnosed pain, a nagging cough, a new restlessness — were probably drawn by the promising title of my book. Some of you may enjoy reading about medical subjects of any kind. Some of you may see doctors fairly regularly, and some of you may resist going to see a doctor until you absolutely must. But the fact that you are reading this book very likely indicates that you are in a position — by virtue of your education — to take advantage of the suggestions I have made. For that reason, I am going to impose a bit longer to remind you about some essential principles of good health.

I am now seventy-six years old and despite my medical history, I feel that I am in good health. I haven't always been in good health. I have had two heart attacks — one in 1984 and another in 1992. It was not until my second heart attack that I woke up and began to listen to my personal physician. I finally saw how unhealthy I was living. I had stopped smoking cigarettes in 1977, thank goodness, but I still was too fat, had high blood pressure, did not exercise, and had high cholesterol. I joined a cardiac rehab program. I knew I had to do some changing. That was sixteen years ago.

Of all the things I considered and did to improve my health, I firmly believe exercise is the most important change I made. By walking briskly every day on a treadmill, I lost forty pounds over a two-year period. I take two pills for high blood pressure and one for cholesterol and one aspirin. My blood pressure and cholesterol are now in the low normal range.

I have found there are three components to exercise that are mandatory if you wish to optimize your health. Exercise is best when it optimizes your aerobic condition, your joint flexibility, and your muscle strength. You must attend to each of these, daily if you can, but at least five days a week. If you can afford to do so, joining a health club will help you get supervision of your exercise program. Exercise experts can help you devise a safe exercise program that will address your aerobic condition, flexibility, and muscle strength. Some businesses now sponsor employee exercise programs because they recognize how important exercise is to employee health. If you cannot afford a health club, or your employer does not provide any kind of health facility, then begin exercising on your own. Simply increasing the distance you walk each day will be a good start, and the public library will provide you with resources on exercises that improve flexibility and strength. Don't say you don't "have time" to exercise. Even if you feel "too tired," find a way. Regular exercise will fairly quickly help you to sleep better and feel less tired. Safe, regular exercise provides the closest thing there is to a panacea. It's the one "cure-all" I endorse.

You may notice I have not mentioned diet. Of course, reducing calories will lead to weight loss, but studies show that the loss will not be maintained with dieting alone. Witness the large profitable weight loss programs that depend on repeated return enrollment. You cannot sustain weight loss unless you burn it off with exercise and keep on exercising. I promise you if you really learn how much walking it takes to burn 100 calories, you will begin to think twice before you eat anything extra. Exercise, exercise, exercise.

There is one other general principle you need to consider. I will call it attention to your relaxation. Each day as we live and work, our bodies become tense and not relaxed. At least once a day, you need to stop and sit and do nothing, and I mean nothing. This period needs to last at least twenty minutes. You can call it meditation, which I prefer, or you can call it prayer or reflection or mindfulness or just relaxation. Whatever you call it, learn to evacuate your mind and just let thoughts drift in and out of consciousness. If you have a religious bent, remember what the Trappist monks say: "God's first language is silence." Be silent to yourself. This silent period will reset your body to a relaxed state.

During these twenty minutes, your body and mind come to their natural resting place. Your blood pressure will come down. Your breathing rate will slow. All sorts of adjustments to your body will occur.

I have one final word on health and living. From my reading I have found that the average human life span is fixed at eighty-five plus or minus five years. The life span for dogs, for comparison, is around twelve years; tortoises can survive for nearly two hundred years. Only a few people live past ninety years. Most reports of extremely long lives have been shown to be falsehoods. If you make it to a hundred, you get your picture on the *Today Show* on TV. Read the obituaries and note how few people are in their nineties. Despite popular notions, the human life span has not increased in recorded history. It is the limit in years for our species, and unless some miraculous alteration of the human genome occurs we will, most of us, live no longer than eighty to ninety years.

There is great confusion between life expectancy from birth and human life span. Life expectancy is the average age at death for the population born in any given year. It has increased from around forty-five years in 1900 to nearly eighty years now. Almost all of the increase in life expectancy from birth is the result of public health measures, such as cleaning up the water and milk supply and vaccination for childhood infectious diseases. These measures have nearly eliminated infant and early childhood death, adding many years to the calculated life expectancy. Medical care, despite popular notions, has had very little or no effect on life expectancy from birth.

In 1900, the life expectancy for an eighty-five-year-old person was about one-and-a-half years. Around 2000, it was only about two-and-a-half years. Medical advances allow more people to survive into their seventies and eighties, but it has not extended the human life span.

What does this mean about you? Here is how I see it. You cannot extend the human life span, but you may be able to add years to your own life expectancy. You certainly can do things to keep yourself in more vigorous condition so that you live more actively in your later years. As someone said, "If I knew I was going to live this long, I would have taken better care of myself." The comedian George Burns, when he was in his nineties, said, "Just don't ever start taking those short steps." Short steps come from loss of joint flexibility and muscular disuse. If you are already taking short steps, start doing stretching exercises or join a yoga class. Work on taking longer steps. Much of what we call aging is simply disuse or "no use" of our bodies. "What you don't use, you lose."

If you are abusing your health by smoking, through excessive alcohol use, overeating, or lack of exercise, you can add years to your life by changing your unhealthy habits. If you are not guilty of unhealthy habits, you can improve your health with regular, daily exercise. And if you are having some symptom, seeking medical advice and following the steps in this book may lead you to the cause.

Remember that even healthy people sometimes develop aches and pains or more seriously troubling symptoms, and that is when you need to ask yourself these questions:

What am I doing in my life that I should not be doing?
What am I not doing in my life that I should be doing?

The answer will often be something you can change.

Appendix I

Some Diagnoses You Never Want Missed

As I said earlier, and want to stress again, modern medicine is extremely good at finding disease. Improvements in testing and screening and new understandings of genetic markers have all helped to increase the speed and reliability of the diagnostic process. However, there are a few diagnoses that can slip through the cracks and there are some curable or treatable diseases that you do not want your physician to miss.

Some diseases can be silent for long periods, or they can produce a variety of symptoms. For a diagnosis to be missed, one of several things will probably be happening:

+ + +

1. The symptoms of the disease may not be localized to an organ system.

They are diffuse and generalized, such as weakness, fatigue, lack of energy, or dizziness. It is difficult for physicians to think of every single disease that is systemic or generalized.

+ + +

2. The disease may be extremely rare and therefore not considered by the doctor in the early list of possibilities.

The doctor must think of the disease and look for it before it can be diagnosed. The following are all rare diseases that can be missed. All of them are also treatable or curable.

Addison's Disease (adrenal failure and lack of cortisol)

<u>Symptoms</u>: Loss of weight, weakness, low blood pressure, and darkening of the skin. Treated by giving daily cortisol replacement.

Hypopituitarism (failure of the pituitary gland with loss of thyroid, adrenal function, and sex hormones)
<u>Symptoms</u>: Weakness, low blood pressure, intolerance to cold temperatures, coarsening of skin, lack of appetite, absence of menses in women, or lack of libido and impotence in men. Treated by replacement of thyroid, adrenal, and gender-appropriate sex hormones.

Hyperparathyroidism (due to small tumor in the parathyroid gland in the neck with high blood calcium and low phosphate levels)
<u>Symptoms</u>: No symptoms for many years, then kidney stones, lack of appetite, abdominal pains, and fragile bones. Cured by surgical removal of the parathyroid tumor.

Pheochromacytoma (high adrenalin levels from an adrenal tumor)
<u>Symptoms</u>: Few symptoms except those related to high blood pressure with wide fluctuations. Cured by surgical removal of the adrenal gland tumor.

Chronic meningitis, fungal or tuberculosis (chronic infection of the brain)
<u>Symptoms</u>: Chronic headaches, fever, general feeling of ill health. Cured by appropriate antibiotics.

Myasthenia gravis
<u>Symptoms</u>: Muscle weakness in any part of the body, double vision, difficulty opening eyes widely. Symptoms are relieved immediately by a test with Intravenous Tensilon. Many drugs can control this condition.

Hemachromatosis (high iron levels as a cause of cirrhosis of the liver)

Symptoms: No symptoms until late in course of the disease when diabetes mellitus and liver failure can occur. Skin is sometimes bronzed. Testing of iron levels needed for anyone with liver disease and diabetes mellitus. Disease is treated by repeated removal of blood.

Wilson's Disease (high copper levels as a cause of acute liver failure)

Symptoms: This disease runs in families. No symptoms until liver failure occurs. Curious rings are visible around the cornea of the eye. Must think of the disease to make a diagnosis early in its course. Disease is treated by drugs that remove copper from the body.

+   +   +

3. The disease is common, and treatable or curable, but the manifestation is rare.

There is an old saying: "Rare manifestations of common diseases are more common than common manifestations of rare diseases." Here are some rare or unusual manifestations of some diseases:

Pericardial effusion in hypothyroidism (fluid collection around the heart)

Symptoms: All of the symptoms of low thyroid function— cold intolerance, coarse skin, feelings of no energy, slow mental functions. The finding of fluid around the heart diverts attention of the physician erroneously to the heart and away from thinking of low thyroid function.

Congestive heart failure (high output) due to peripheral arterio-venous fistula.

Symptoms: All of the symptoms of congestive heart failure — edema of legs, shortness of breath, no energy, weakness. The presence of a previous traumatic injury, such as a stabbing or gunshot wound, can create large blood flows through an artery to vein connection (AV fistula) and lead to heart failure. Surgical repair of the vascular connection can cure the heart failure.

Congestive heart failure (high output, in hyperthyroidism). Another curable form of heart failure.

Symptoms: All of the symptoms of congestive heart failure with edema of the legs, enlarged heart, shortness of breath, no energy, and weakness. High thyroid blood levels can produce heart failure. Treatment of the hyperthyroidism will cure the heart failure.

+   +   +

4. The abnormal finding on physical examination is missed.

Here are some conditions that can be easily missed on physical examination. Again, all of these conditions are curable or treatable.

Aortic insufficiency (very faint murmur)
Mitral stenosis (murmur is very localized to a small area)
Pulmonary stenosis (faint murmur)
Tumor inside the atrium of the heart (a changing murmur that mimics the sounds of mitral insufficiency)

Symptoms: These four conditions, early on, have no symptoms. Eventually, unless found and surgically corrected, all lead to heart failure. They must be listened for by the physician. I list them here because the murmurs are faint and difficult to hear.

The physician must "think" of these conditions and listen carefully to hear the characteristic sounds.

Coarctation of the aorta with hypertension (absent pulses at the ankle)

Symptoms: There are no symptoms until late in the course. A coarctation is a narrowing of the aorta. This narrowing causes very high blood pressures in the arms and low blood pressure in the legs. It is a known cause of high blood pressure and can be surgically corrected. Everyone with high blood pressure needs to have the blood pressure measured in the legs to detect this disorder.

+   +   +

The diagnoses listed here make up my list of treatable diseases that I never want to miss in any patient I see. Some of these conditions will be asymptomatic for a long period. Before you spend a lot of time with diary keeping or seeking other causes for your puzzling symptoms, be sure your doctor has ruled out all of these and other treatable diseases.

Appendix II

MAST: A Diagnostic Test for Alcoholism

Michigan Alcoholism Screening Test (MAST) Circle any YES answer

1. Do you feel you are a normal drinker? (Normal means you drink less than or as much as other people and you have not developed recurring trouble while drinking.)

2. Have you ever awakened the morning after some drinking the night before and found that you could not remember part of the evening?

3. Do you, your parents, any other near relative, your spouse, or any girlfriend or boyfriend ever worry or complain about your drinking?

4. Can you stop drinking without a struggle after one or two drinks?

5. Do you feel guilty about your drinking?

6. Do friends or relatives think you are a normal drinker?

7. Are you able to stop drinking when you want to?

8. Have you ever attended a meeting of Alcoholics Anonymous (AA)?

9. Have you been in physical fights when you have been drinking?

10. Has your drinking ever created problems between you and either your parents, another relative, your spouse, or any girlfriend or boyfriend?

11. Has any family member of yours ever gone to anyone for help about your drinking?

12. Have you ever lost friends because of drinking?

13. Have you ever been in trouble at work or at school because of drinking?

14. Have you ever lost a job because of drinking?

15. Have you ever neglected your obligations, your school work, your family, or your job for two or more days in a row because you were drinking?

16. Do you drink before noon fairly often?

17. Have you ever been told you have liver trouble or cirrhosis?

18. After heavy drinking, have you ever had severe shaking, or heard voices or seen things that were not really there?

19. Have you ever gone to anyone for help about your drinking?

20. Have you ever been in a hospital because of drinking?

21. Have you ever been a patient in a psychiatric hospital or on a psychiatric ward of a general hospital where

drinking was part of the problem that resulted in your hospitalization?

22. Have you ever been seen at a psychiatric or mental health clinic or gone to any doctor, social worker, or clergy for help with any emotional problem where drinking was part of the problem?

23. Have you ever been arrested for drunk driving, driving while intoxicated, or driving under the influence of alcoholic beverages or any other drug? (If yes, how many times?)

24. Have you ever been arrested or taken into custody, even for a few hours, because of drunken behavior?

Key to the MAST Test
Answer For Each Question - Score Points
In The Following Fashion:

1.   2 for No
2.   2 for Yes
3.   1 for Yes
4.   2 for No
5.   1 for Yes
6.   2 for No
7.   2 for No
8.   5 for Yes
9.   1 for Yes
10.   2 for Yes
11.   2 for Yes
12.   2 for Yes
13.   2 for Yes
14.   2 for Yes
15.   2 for Yes
16.   1 for Yes
17.   2 for Yes
18.   2 for Yes
19.   5 for Yes
20.   5 for Yes
21.   2 for Yes
22.   2 for Yes
23.   2 for Yes
24.   2 for Yes

Score 5 points for hallucinations or delirium tremens and score 2 points for each additional episode experienced.

Interpretation:

0-3 points = probably normal drinker

4 points = borderline score

5-9 points = 80% associated with alcoholism/chemical
dependence

10 or more points = 100% associated with alcoholism

Dr. Anderson Spickard, Jr. (Anderson Spickard, Jr., M.D. and Barbara R. Thompson; Nashville, TN: *Dying for a Drink*, W Publishing Company, Thomas Nelson, 2005) uses the scores in the following manner: Quoting him, "If the score is 10-15, I am comfortable with recommending the patient attend Alcoholics Anonymous meetings regularly. If the score is higher, in the range of 15-20, it is unlikely that AA meetings are enough for the patient, and I recommend inpatient or intensive outpatient treatment after she or he is detoxified."

Appendix III

Format for Diary for Recording Symptoms
Step One: Record Score of Symptoms

Time	Sun	Mon	Tues	Wed	Thurs	Fri	Sat
2:00 a.m.							
4:00 a.m.							
6:00 a.m.							
8:00 a.m.							
10:00 a.m.							
12:00 noon							
2:00 p.m.							
4:00 p.m.							
6:00 p.m.							
8:00 p.m.							
10:00 p.m.							
12:00 midnight							

Step One:

In each blank, insert the intensity score of your symptoms (on a scale of 0 to 10). Only record scores at night if you wake up. Record your symptom scores for an entire week.

You are looking for variations or the "wobbles" of your symptoms by the time of day or day of the week.

What is the pattern of your symptom?

Appendix III

Format for Diary for Recording Symptoms
Step Two: Making Observations

Day of Week:_____   Date:_____

Time	Location	Symptom Score	Observations
6 a.m.- 12 noon			Air*_____ Oral*_____ Skin*_____ Social* _____ Other:
12 noon- 6 p.m.			Air: _____ Oral: _____ Skin: _____ Social: _____ Other:
6 p.m.- 12 midnight			Air: _____ Oral: _____ Skin: _____ Social: _____ Other:
12 midnight- 6 a.m.			Air: _____ Oral: _____ Skin: _____ Social: _____ Other:

Suggested Observations

*Air and Surroundings	*Oral Intake	*Skin Contacts	*Social Setting and People
Indoors	Drugs (list)	Cosmetics	People Present
Outdoors	Food	Soap	Conversation Topics
Dust or Pollen	Liquids	Laundry Detergent	In-laws
Air or Heating Vent	Toothpaste	Clothing	People in Thoughts
Location	Mouthwashes	Jewelry	Memories
Animals and Pets	Other	Other	Dreams
Plants			Other
Other			

Step Two: (Use a separate page for each day of the week)
Using the information from Step One, begin to make observations for the time period preceding the intense symptom. Pay attention to substances, people, and your surroundings. Ask yourself:

What am I doing in my life that I should not be doing?

What am I not doing in my life that I should be doing?

Appendix III

Format for Diary for Recording Symptoms
Step Two: Making Observations

Day of Week:_____   Date:_____

Time	Location	Symptom Score	Observations
6 a.m.- 12 noon			Air*_____ Oral*_____ Skin*_____ Social*_____ Other:
12 noon- 6 p.m.			Air: _____ Oral: _____ Skin: _____ Social: _____ Other:
6 p.m.- 12 midnight			Air: _____ Oral: _____ Skin:_____ Social: _____ Other:
12 midnight- 6 a.m.			Air: _____ Oral: _____ Skin: _____ Social: _____ Other:

Suggested Observations

*Air and Surroundings	*Oral Intake	*Skin Contacts	*Social Setting and People
Indoors	Drugs (list)	Cosmetics	People Present
Outdoors	Food	Soap	Conversation Topics
Dust or Pollen	Liquids	Laundry Detergent	In-laws
Air or Heating Vent	Toothpaste	Clothing	People in Thoughts
Location	Mouthwashes	Jewelry	Memories
Animals and Pets	Other	Other	Dreams
Plants			Other
Other			

Step Two: (Use a separate page for each day of the week)
Using the information from Step One, begin to make observations for the time period preceding the intense symptom. Pay attention to substances, people, and your surroundings. Ask yourself:

What am I doing in my life that I should not be doing?

What am I not doing in my life that I should be doing?

Appendix III

Format for Diary for Recording Symptoms
Step Two: Making Observations

Day of Week:_____   Date:_____

Time	Location	Symptom Score	Observations
6 a.m.- 12 noon			Air*_____ Oral*_____ Skin*_____ Social*_____ Other:
12 noon- 6 p.m.			Air: _____ Oral: _____ Skin:_____ Social: _____ Other:
6 p.m.- 12 midnight			Air: _____ Oral: _____ Skin:_____ Social: _____ Other:
12 midnight- 6 a.m.			Air: _____ Oral: _____ Skin:_____ Social: _____ Other:

Suggested Observations

*Air and Surroundings	*Oral Intake	*Skin Contacts	*Social Setting and People
Indoors	Drugs (list)	Cosmetics	People Present
Outdoors	Food	Soap	Conversation Topics
Dust or Pollen	Liquids	Laundry Detergent	In-laws
Air or Heating Vent	Toothpaste	Clothing	People in Thoughts
Location	Mouthwashes	Jewelry	Memories
Animals and Pets	Other	Other	Dreams
Plants			Other
Other			

Step Two: (Use a separate page for each day of the week)
Using the information from Step One, begin to make observations for the time period preceding the intense symptom. Pay attention to substances, people, and your surroundings. Ask yourself:

What am I doing in my life that I should not be doing?

What am I not doing in my life that I should be doing?

Appendix III

Format for Diary for Recording Symptoms
Step Two: Making Observations

Day of Week:_____   Date:_____

Time	Location	Symptom Score	Observations
6 a.m.- 12 noon			Air*_____ Oral*_____ Skin*_____ Social* _____ Other:
12 noon- 6 p.m.			Air: _____ Oral: _____ Skin:_____ Social: _____ Other:
6 p.m.- 12 midnight			Air: _____ Oral: _____ Skin:_____ Social: _____ Other:
12 midnight- 6 a.m.			Air: _____ Oral: _____ Skin:_____ Social: _____ Other:

Suggested Observations

*Air and Surroundings	*Oral Intake	*Skin Contacts	*Social Setting and People
Indoors	Drugs (list)	Cosmetics	People Present
Outdoors	Food	Soap	Conversation Topics
Dust or Pollen	Liquids	Laundry Detergent	In-laws
Air or Heating Vent	Toothpaste	Clothing	People in Thoughts
Location	Mouthwashes	Jewelry	Memories
Animals and Pets	Other	Other	Dreams
Plants			Other
Other			

Step Two: (Use a separate page for each day of the week)
Using the information from Step One, begin to make observations for the time period preceding the intense symptom. Pay attention to substances, people, and your surroundings. Ask yourself:

What am I doing in my life that I should not be doing?

What am I not doing in my life that I should be doing?

Appendix III

Format for Diary for Recording Symptoms
Step Two: Making Observations

Day of Week:_____   Date:_____

Time	Location	Symptom Score	Observations
6 a.m.- 12 noon			Air*_____ Oral*_____ Skin*_____ Social* _____ Other:
12 noon- 6 p.m.			Air: _____ Oral: _____ Skin: _____ Social: _____ Other:
6 p.m.- 12 midnight			Air: _____ Oral: _____ Skin: _____ Social: _____ Other:
12 midnight- 6 a.m.			Air: _____ Oral: _____ Skin: _____ Social: _____ Other:

Suggested Observations

*Air and Surroundings	*Oral Intake	*Skin Contacts	*Social Setting and People
Indoors	Drugs (list)	Cosmetics	People Present
Outdoors	Food	Soap	Conversation Topics
Dust or Pollen	Liquids	Laundry Detergent	In-laws
Air or Heating Vent	Toothpaste	Clothing	People in Thoughts
Location	Mouthwashes	Jewelry	Memories
Animals and Pets	Other	Other	Dreams
Plants			Other
Other			

Step Two: (Use a separate page for each day of the week)
Using the information from Step One, begin to make observations for the time period preceding the intense symptom. Pay attention to substances, people, and your surroundings. Ask yourself:

What am I doing in my life that I should not be doing?

What am I not doing in my life that I should be doing?

Appendix III

Format for Diary for Recording Symptoms
Step Two: Making Observations

Day of Week:_____   Date:_____

Time	Location	Symptom Score	Observations
6 a.m.- 12 noon			Air*_____ Oral*_____ Skin*_____ Social*_____ Other:
12 noon- 6 p.m.			Air: _____ Oral: _____ Skin:_____ Social: _____ Other:
6 p.m.- 12 midnight			Air: _____ Oral: _____ Skin:_____ Social: _____ Other:
12 midnight- 6 a.m.			Air: _____ Oral: _____ Skin:_____ Social: _____ Other:

Suggested Observations

*Air and Surroundings	*Oral Intake	*Skin Contacts	*Social Setting and People
Indoors	Drugs (list)	Cosmetics	People Present
Outdoors	Food	Soap	Conversation Topics
Dust or Pollen	Liquids	Laundry Detergent	In-laws
Air or Heating Vent	Toothpaste	Clothing	People in Thoughts
Location	Mouthwashes	Jewelry	Memories
Animals and Pets	Other	Other	Dreams
Plants			Other
Other			

Step Two: (Use a separate page for each day of the week)
Using the information from Step One, begin to make observations for the time period preceding the intense symptom. Pay attention to substances, people, and your surroundings. Ask yourself:

What am I doing in my life that I should not be doing?

What am I not doing in my life that I should be doing?

Appendix III

Format for Diary for Recording Symptoms
Step Two: Making Observations

Day of Week:_____   Date:_____

Time	Location	Symptom Score	Observations
6 a.m.- 12 noon			Air*_____ Oral*_____ Skin*_____ Social*_____ Other:
12 noon- 6 p.m.			Air: _____ Oral: _____ Skin: _____ Social: _____ Other:
6 p.m.- 12 midnight			Air: _____ Oral: _____ Skin: _____ Social: _____ Other:
12 midnight- 6 a.m.			Air: _____ Oral: _____ Skin: _____ Social: _____ Other:

Suggested Observations

*Air and Surroundings	*Oral Intake	*Skin Contacts	*Social Setting and People
Indoors	Drugs (list)	Cosmetics	People Present
Outdoors	Food	Soap	Conversation Topics
Dust or Pollen	Liquids	Laundry Detergent	In-laws
Air or Heating Vent	Toothpaste	Clothing	People in Thoughts
Location	Mouthwashes	Jewelry	Memories
Animals and Pets	Other	Other	Dreams
Plants			Other
Other			

Step Two: (Use a separate page for each day of the week)
Using the information from Step One, begin to make observations for the time period preceding the intense symptom. Pay attention to substances, people, and your surroundings. Ask yourself:

What am I doing in my life that I should not be doing?
What am I not doing in my life that I should be doing?

Appendix IV

Share Your Experiences and Success with Others

Many of you have experienced success in relieving your symptoms with the methods and information described in *Puzzling Symptoms*. We want to hear from you and ask that you share your story with others. You may or may not give us your name. Your story may help someone who is still symptomatic under a similar circumstance. (Use additional pages as necessary.)

Provide a brief story of your symptoms:

_____

_____

_____

Describe how you uncovered the cause of your symptoms:

_____

_____

_____

Describe what you did to obtain relief or improvement in your symptoms:

_____

_____

_____

❑ You have permission to publish my story but *do not* use my name:

Sign:_____Date: _____

May we contact you if necessary?   ❑ Yes ❑ No

❑ Yes, you have permission to publish my story and use my name:

Sign:_____Date: _____

Please print your name: _____

Age _____   ❑ Male   ❑ Female

Address: _____

City_____ State: ___ Zip:_____ Phone: _____

E-mail:_____

Mail this form to: Cable Publishing, Attn: Puzzling Symptoms Reports, 14090 E. Keinenen Road, Brule, WI 54820

Fax this form to: 715-372-8448

About the Author

Dr. Clifton K. Meador, born in Alabama in 1931, attended Vanderbilt School of Medicine in Nashville where he graduated with top honors. He completed his internship and began his residency at Columbia Presbyterian Hospital in New York, then spent two years in the Army Medical Corps before completing his residency and N.I.H. Fellowship in Endocrinology at Vanderbilt.

During his long and varied medical career, Dr. Meador directed the N.I.H. Clinical Research Center in Alabama, served as dean of the School of Medicine at the University of Alabama in Birmingham, created the Vanderbilt teaching service at Saint Thomas Hospital in Nashville, Tennessee, and trained young doctors as Professor of Medicine at Vanderbilt University and Meharry Medical College. For the past ten years, he has served as Executive Director of the Meharry Vanderbilt Alliance, a foundation that supports a collaborative clinical, educational, research, and training program for Meharry Medical College and Vanderbilt University.

Dr. Meador has published extensively in medical literature; he is perhaps best known for "The Art and Science of Nondisease" and "The Last Well Person," both published in the *New England Journal of Medicine*, and "A Lament for Invalids," published in the *Journal of the American Medical Association*. The articles are satiric treatments of the excesses of medical practice.

Dr. Meador is the author of many popular medical books, including *Symptoms of Unknown Origin*, *Little Book of Doctor's Rules*, *Little Book of Nurse's Rules*, and *Med School*. He enjoys woodworking and furniture making, golf (a goal is to shoot his age), and his favorite hobby — writing. Meador is the proud father of seven children. He is married to Ann Cowden, an accomplished portrait artist.

Other Books by Clifton K. Meador, M.D.

A Little Book of Doctors' Rules,[*] by Clifton K. Meador, M.D., Philadelphia, PA: Hanley and Belfus, 1992.

A Little Book of Nurses' Rules, by Rosalie Hammerschmidt, R.N., and Clifton K. Meador, M.D., Philadelphia, PA: Hanley and Belfus, 1993.

Pearls from a Pediatric Practice I, by William Wadlington, M.D., and Clifton K. Meador, M.D., Philadelphia, PA: Hanley and Belfus, 1998.

A Little Book of Doctors' Rules II: A Compilation, by Clifton K. Meador, M.D., Philadelphia, PA: Hanley and Belfus, 1999.

A Little Book of Emergency Medicine Rules, by Corey M. Slovis, M.D., Keith D. Wrenn, M.D., and Clifton K. Meador, M.D., Philadelphia, PA: Hanley and Belfus, 2000.

How to Raise Healthy and Happy Children: A Pediatrician's Pearls for Parents, by William Wadlington, M.D., Clifton K. Meador, M.D., and Marietta Howington, M.A., Authors Choice Press, iUniverse.com, Inc., 2001.

The Unknown Woman and Her Children: The Meador Family of Myrtlewood, by Clifton K. Meador, Privately Published, 1995.

Symptoms of Unknown Origin: A Medical Odyssey, by Clifton K. Meador, M.D., Nashville, TN: Vanderbilt University Press, 2005.

Twentieth Century Men in Medicine: Personal Reflections, by Clifton K Meador, M.D., Authors Choice Press, iUniverse.com, Inc., 2007.

Med School, A new edition, by Clifton K. Meador, M.D., Brule, WI: Cable Publishing, 2008.

*Translated into Japanese, Spanish, Polish, Italian, and Indonesian.

Puzzling Symptoms
Order Form

Fax orders: 715-372-8448

Telephone orders: 715-372-8499

Website orders: www.cablepublishing.com

E-mail orders: nan@cablepublishing.com

Postal orders: Cable Publishing
14090 E Keinenen Rd.
Brule, WI 54820

Name:_____

Address:_____

City:_____ State:_____ Zip:_____

Telephone:_____

E-mail address:_____

_____ **Number of copies** at $12.95 each $_____

Sales tax: Please add 5.5% for Wisconsin addresses _____

Shipping: _____
   ($3.50 for the first book, $.50 for each additional book)

Total order: $_____

Payment: ___Check or ___Visa ___MC ___AMEX ___Discover

Card number: _____

Name on card:_____ Exp.date:_____